Principles of
Day Surgery Nursing

Also of interest:

Blackwell Science, in consultation with Moira Edmondson and Gobnait Waters, have produced Day Surgery *Server*.

Day Surgery *Server* is a unique information management system, specifically designed to deliver a high-quality, comprehensive service to patients which streamlines the day-to-day running of the day surgery department, from pre-operative assessment to discharge. The system directly addresses the problems of providing adequate information for patients (pre- and post-procedure), contract monitoring and waiting list management. The emphasis of Day Surgery *Server* is on patient care, patient communication and quality control, and can easily be customised to suit individual unit requirements.

For further information, please contact:

Day Surgery *Server*
Blackwell Science Ltd
Osney Mead
Oxford OX2 0EL
UK

Principles of
Day Surgery Nursing

Sarah Penn RGN
*President of British Association of Day Surgery
Manager, Day Surgery Unit,
Addenbrooke's NHS Trust, Cambridge*

Harold T. Davenport FRCPC, FFARCS
*Honorary Consultant Anaesthetist,
Northwick Park and St Mark's NHS Trust
Honorary Editor of Journal of One-Day Surgery*

Susan Carrington RGN, CMS, CM
*Collection Manager for the Midlands and South West Zone,
The National Blood Service
Formerly Manager, UBHT Day Surgery Unit, Bristol*

Moira Edmondson RGN, MBSR
*Director of Day Surgery and Private Patient Services,
Kent and Canterbury Hospitals NHS Trust*

Blackwell
Science

© 1996 by Blackwell Science Ltd,
a Blackwell Publishing Company
Editorial Offices:
Osney Mead, Oxford OX2 0EL, UK
  Tel: +44 (0)1865 206206
Blackwell Science, Inc., 350 Main Street,
Malden, MA 02148-5018, USA
  Tel: +1 781 388 8250
Iowa State Press, a Blackwell Publishing
Company, 2121 State Avenue, Ames, Iowa
50014-8300, USA
  Tel: +1 515 292 0140
Blackwell Publishing Asia Pty Ltd,
550 Swanston Street, Carlton South,
Melbourne, Victoria 3053, Australia
  Tel: +61 (0)3 9347 0300
Blackwell Wissenschafts Verlag,
Kurfürstendamm 57, 10707 Berlin, Germany
  Tel: +49 (0)30 32 79 060

First published 1996
Reprinted 2003

Library of Congress
Cataloging-in-Publication Data

Principles of day surgery nursing/Sara Penn
  ... [et al.].
    p. cm.
  Includes bibliographical references and
index.
  ISBN 0-632-03973-6 (pbk.)
  1. Ambulatory surgical nursing. I. Penn,
Sarah.
  [DNLM: 1. Ambulatory Surgery —
nursing. WY 161 P9565 1996]
RD110.5.P76 1996
610.73'677 — dc20
DNLM/DLC
for Library of Congress   96-34126
                                       CIP

ISBN 0-632-03973-6

A catalogue record for this title is available
from the British Library

Set in 10/12pt Palatino
by DP Photosetting, Aylesbury, Bucks
Printed and bound in Great Britain by
Marston Lindsay Ross International Ltd,
Oxfordshire

For further information on
Blackwell Publishing, visit our website:
www.blackwellpublishing.com

Contents

Foreword

Whatever the prevailing system of social security, the burden of health costs on public finances and on the resources of individuals continues to grow by orders of magnitude that are difficult to sustain. Available resources and the full capacity of the strongest interventions must be committed to the cases that require them. To complain that resources are scarce is unacceptable as long as responsible use is not being made of those already available.

Thanks to modern techniques, to new medicines, and to adapted structures, day surgery can make a powerful contribution – and to the complete satisfaction of patients, doctors and nurses. Guaranteeing high quality care for all citizens of our countries is now a major challenge for society. Day surgery provides an exceptional opportunity to meet this challenge. Indeed, compared with proposals generally focused on managing shortages or restricting access to care, day surgery is one of the rare innovative strategies. To advance day surgery, we must inform, train, educate and mobilise, with commitment and persistence. This is the goal, and indeed the merit of *Principles of Day Surgery Nursing*.

Certainly, day surgery is as old as surgery itself. But what *is* new is the systematised approach of day surgery, that is, the specific organisation and structure that are put in place. Day surgery is not simply an abbreviated hospital stay, but rather a completely original concept: architectural, organisational, therapeutic, economic and qualitative. Fundamentally, organisation is central to the concept of day surgery, and the patient – not the doctor any more – is at the centre of this organisation.

Among the many benefits often quoted to advance the development of day surgery – which include, for example, care that is better adapted to patients who are not ill, absence of nosocomial infection, reduction of psychological stress associated with hospitalisation (especially for children), time savings, and more rapid return to regular life – the improvement of working conditions for nursing staff should be noted in particular.

In many countries, the nursing profession is in crisis. It is rebelling against arduous working conditions and hours (nights and weekends), inadequacy of personnel and resources allotted to it, and low salary levels. These concerns are compounded with those that inevitably flow from normal family obligations for staff that is most often female, resulting in a chronic shortage of nurses.

Working conditions in day surgery units (DSU) are characterised by schedules that are completely compatible with harmonious family life; part-time work can easily be planned; the work is varied and marked with a team spirit that turns to good account the contribution of each actor – and their mutual respect – resulting in successful performance for DSUs.

Thus, vigorous and well-planned development of day hospitalisation can help resolve many of the difficulties of nursing staff, and retain, or bring back to the workplace mothers who are attracted by the kind of working conditions common in DSUs.

Nevertheless, despite the accepted benefits, and the almost universal support for day surgery, it is still advancing much more slowly than should be expected. Unfortunately, time is needed to plan and put into place policies that are truly effective and motivating. And resistance to change is typical of men – and women.

Principles of Day Surgery Nursing aims to promote and develop a high quality of care within day surgery. The authors are tireless pioneers of day surgery, active for many years on all fronts – in practice, management, organisation, education, quality control – and on every scientific and political, national and international stage. We should all be grateful to them.

Dr Cl. De Lathouwer
President, International Association of Ambulatory Surgery

Preface

A new treatment or investigation method can revolutionise medical practice overnight. Changing the manner in which care is provided is usually evolutionary and relatively slow, but the recent rapid growth of day surgery will, in the years to come, change the pattern of health care services markedly. There will be many far-reaching consequences for patients and staff, and the nursing profession must learn to cope with day surgery effectively and efficiently.

Principles of Day Surgery Nursing provides nurses with the information they need to play a major role in the team which organises, manages and runs a day care unit. Because day care practice is both innovative and an exciting challenge, this text is primarily intended to provoke thought and discussion. Nurses' learning and actions are crucial if day surgery is to avoid being a second rate service and one which is provided as a cost cutting exercise. The manner in which nurses practice must support the public's widespread appreciation of and increasing demand for this method of dealing with many of their ills.

As stated in its constitution, a prime objective of the British Association of Day Surgery, a major part of whose membership are nurses, is 'to encourage the expansion of high quality day surgery'. It is our wish that this book will help readers contribute to that objective.

Harold T. Davenport
April 1996

Acknowledgements

We wish to acknowledge, with thanks, the publishers for their editorial assistance in the production of this book and Dr Tom Ogg for his advice.

We mention our special appreciation for the contribution of the cartoons by Emma-Louise Edmondson and Mark Straker.

Our thanks also go to Nigel Penn, Brian Edmondson, Mike Mussen and Margaret Davenport for their support, encouragement and enthusiasm throughout the writing of this book.

Dr Claude De Lathouwer has kindly contributed a foreword.

Chapter 1
The Day Surgery Scene

Harold T. Davenport

Introduction

Day surgery is a new term for an old concept. In the past, hospitals were mainly used by the poor, travellers or sometimes the military until, in the Victorian era, the large voluntary hospitals – which were mainly charitable institutions – and council hospitals were developed. These became more widely used with the introduction of medical insurance and the advent of the National Health Service (NHS), though many rich patients preferred to have their operations in their own home and King George VI had major surgery at Buckingham Palace. When elective operations became more complicated and took more time, and also when the Lister spray control of infection was replaced by asepsis and anaesthesia became more complex, more and more operations were undertaken in hospital, with the patient staying for many days and often weeks afterwards. Even today some older surgeons practise as they were taught and keep patients in a hospital bed for 10–14 days after the repair of an inguinal hernia.

The seminal reports on day surgery were made by a surgeon, James Nicoll, in 1909 and an anaesthetist, Ralph Waters, in 1919 who worked in Glasgow and Sioux City, Iowa respectively. They proposed that chosen operations in children and adults could, and should, be undertaken with patients returning home within a few hours. However, until the last three decades, the structure of health care meant that their pioneering ideas were taken up by only a few enthusiasts. The recent strong impetus to increase day surgery is undoubtedly based on financial considerations.

Nurses have recognised that many patients, after certain surgical operations and particularly with the newer operative techniques and anaesthetics, need little prolonged expert nursing care afterwards. They have become aware, as is shown throughout this book, that a different set of nursing activities and policies are needed if this form of care is to be safe and successful. It is nurses, in the main, who have managed the new day surgery units and they are actively exploring all aspects of day care as it increases in volume and complexity. In Britain, it was originally a few keen surgeons, anaesthetists and nurses who, in that order, fostered day surgery but now it is nurses who are in the vanguard of this revolutionary change in the pattern of medical care.

Such a major reorganisation provides an excellent reason to question old unexamined routines. It also provides an opportunity to study new methods which will benefit in-patients as much as out-patients. Day care appears to be very much the patients' preference, perhaps providentially making the everyday surgery

Table 1.1   Some notable dates in British day surgery history.

1800	Humphrey Davy in Bristol wrote of breathing nitrous oxide: 'It may probably be used with advantage during surgical operations'
	Most nineteenth-century anaesthesia from 1842 was not given in hospitals
1853	John Snow gave Queen Victoria chloroform for home delivery
1853	Alexander Wood invented the syringe and needle in Edinburgh
1899	James Nicoll practised paediatric day surgery with a 'boarding house' in Glasgow
1900	Local and regional block anaesthesia came from Europe
1933	Ronald Jarman reported the use of intravenous barbiturates (Evipan)
1941	Richard Asher wrote a classic article 'The dangers of going to bed'
1951	Rex Lawrie at Guy's hospital espoused more paediatric day surgery
1955	Eric Farquharson reported day care hernia repair in Edinburgh
1961	Hugh Dudley organised intermediate day surgery in Aberdeen
1967	James Calnan used a Quonset hut as an autonomous unit at Hammersmith Hospital (NHS)
1975	Day surgery unit design and function propagated by Tom Ogg and James Burns (Cambridge and Southampton)
1981	Wellington Day-Care Freestanding Unit opened in Harley Street (Humana)
1985	Royal College of Surgeons published guidelines for day case surgery
1990	Government backing of day surgery appeared (NHS and Audit Commission reports)
1990	British Association of Day Surgery was formed
1991	*Journal of One-Day Surgery* was launched
1991	The first hospital 'hotel' opened in Kingston upon Thames
1992	The Audit Commission report on day medicine was published
1993	*Ambulatory Surgery Journal* was launched
1995	First International Congress on Ambulatory Surgery was held in Brussels

unit a 'house of guests' – the Latin derivation of the word 'hospital'. As day care patients, like guests, are independent and responsible for much of their care, the perioperative role of nurses has to be greatly expanded to make this possible.

Present state of development

In recent times, the first hospital-based day care units are claimed by Grand Rapids in 1951 and Los Angeles Hospital in 1952. Then came the free-standing surgicenter in Phoenix in 1969. In the UK, day care units are predominantly within the hospital precinct, whereas in the USA a very large number of free-standing units have been created. When day care units were first organised in the UK, utilisation was extremely variable for a number of reasons. Consultant surgeons, physicians and anaesthetists were reluctant to change their form of practice to one which required more continuous involvement with patients. Day care also required them to be involved in more minor and intermediate procedures which, in the in-patients setting, were often delegated to junior hospital house staff. Bed occupancy statistics, usually taken at midnight, were important to both surgeons and managers as measures of their workload and status, and nurse managers were slow to recognise day care as a major mainstream rather than a minor sideline activity. On the other hand, long waiting lists, shortages of beds and anaesthetists, and now charter standards have stimulated increased day care activity.

By the 1980s there were sufficient active units to explore many clinical, organisational, social and financial aspects of day care work. The results showed that, for certain patients, day surgery was the preferred form of treatment, and in 1985 the Royal College of Surgeons and the government published official guidelines which encouraged an expansion of the proportion of surgery to be done as day work. Both suggested that in most specialities 50% was a realistic target, a figure which had been exceeded elsewhere.

Economic aspects

It is obvious that efficiency is improved if one can avoid two or three nights of costly hospital hotel service when it is not essential for patients undergoing some procedures. The proviso is that carers are available at home and will act without pay. However, arriving at a cost–benefit analysis is extremely complex and present accounting within the NHS is inadequate for the task.

The key features for an economic study are:

(1) When the patient goes home, extra or new services are required in the community, but this is not as costly as an in-patient bed service. Nevertheless, average in-patient cost provides an inaccurate guide comparison because the actual day of an operation is the most expensive.

(2) In a hospital an empty bed represents a saving of only 20% of total cost (this does not apply to free-standing day care units) because fixed costs of the buildings must still be borne. To recognise the full saving of day care, buildings have to be closed down.

(3) Five-day nursing, without unsocial hours and weekend payments, markedly reduces the 'daily average cost' but the day care unit must be fully utilised. This ideally should include out-of-hours use for general practitioner surgery, sterilisations (male and female), evening assessment and pain clinics, plus educational renting, such as Red Cross classes.

(4) Major cost savings have arisen by the elimination of routine pre-operative investigations, clinical examinations and voluminous documentation.

(5) The capital costs of building a day care unit are considerable, and tend to be greater for conversion than building new. Costs must include equipment because borrowing or transfer from other areas is rarely satisfactory.

A recent report published by the University of Ottawa in Canada, using costings from an advanced database at the University of Alberta, showed that in-patient care was three times more costly than day surgery. Of course, many studies show there are considerable differences in case-mixed groups – in Alberta the day surgery saving per case ranged from $342 for hernia repair to $754 for knee procedures. In this study re-admission and home care costs were not considered significant overall. Future cost savings which should be explored are those involving staffing – the major element of all health care costs – and could entail a wide use of assistants and operating department practitioners trained specifically for day care, part-time early retired consultants and specialists, and trained general practitioners. However, increasing the less-qualified staff can undermine the service quality dangerously, with minimal cost savings. Volunteers may also be attracted into the friendly circumscribed milieu of a day surgery unit which is not as intimidating to them as a major hospital may be.

Design and ambience

The Department of Health has recently updated its building notes on accommodation for day care. Building Note number 52 is in three parts: (1) Day Surgery Unit; (2) Endoscopy Unit; and (3) Medical Investigation and Treatment Unit. These and other government publications are essential for any planning to ensure statutory regulations are complied with. Plans must embody such objects as fire protection, sanitation and parking laws.

The government notes are meant as a guide for district general hospitals but each location will have its own particular needs and case mix which will dictate the type of unit required. It is wasteful and time-consuming for every different project team to agonise over design when adjustment of standard units, modified by feedback from previous users, can be utilised. Because of the projected increase in the growth of day care it is crucial that future expansion should be allowed for in all plans.

Patients find it more convenient if the day care unit is at ground level with easy access and adjacent parking. Parking problems are one of the main dissatisfactions expressed by patients attending day care units and where planning is for the unit to occupy a 'green field site', ideally one third of the area should be available for parking and another third for landscaping. Units should aim to be as unhospital-like and as informal as possible, and the surroundings are important in that respect for the comfort of waiting patients.

Internally the decor and furnishing, by appropriate use of fabrics, colours, lighting and scheming, can be pleasurable for patients and staff. The flow of patients through a unit should be as logical as possible, and in particular the reception area must be welcoming, quiet and uncrowded. Integrated operating theatres should be identical to those in any general hospital so that the unit is prepared if emergency surgery is required, or if the type of surgery to be covered by the unit becomes more major. The continuous pre-preparation, operation, recovery and ward areas require changing and toilet facilities for staff and patients, and it is important that office, waiting, teaching and consultation space is provided. Anaesthetic rooms, primary recovery areas and kitchens may not be considered vital but as day surgery is likely to expand, they would be advisable.

The use of up-to-date means for internal and external communication will save considerable time and effort, so advanced information technology should be an integral part of the planning, where possible. With such communications the X-ray and pathology departments may not need to be adjacent to the day care unit. Security for day units also needs special arrangements as there has to be free access in working hours but security against vandals when closed. Finally, there must be suitable access and toilet structures for children, the disabled and older people, otherwise they will be poorly served or excluded.

Infection control

The purpose of infection control in the day surgery setting is to prevent the occurrence of infections. This may appear to be stating the obvious but the standards of infection control in the theatres and all areas throughout the unit must be no different from those in the rest of the hospital. All users of the unit bear some responsibility for maintaining standards. Written policies and procedures must be formulated and implemented, and an infection control or health and safety group must be convened. The purpose of this group is to implement the policies and procedures maintained in the hospital as a whole as well as those that are specific to day care.

For the patient, any infection will delay recovery and cause unnecessary stress. As the patient's experience of day surgery is very short (where the majority do not require out-patient follow-up), robust practices and audit methods must be in place to ensure that any infection post-discharge can be recorded and correlated. More importantly, measures must be taken subsequently to address the source of any problem that is identified.

Hygiene

Personal cleanliness of patients and staff is of great importance. Patients should be given written instructions regarding bathing

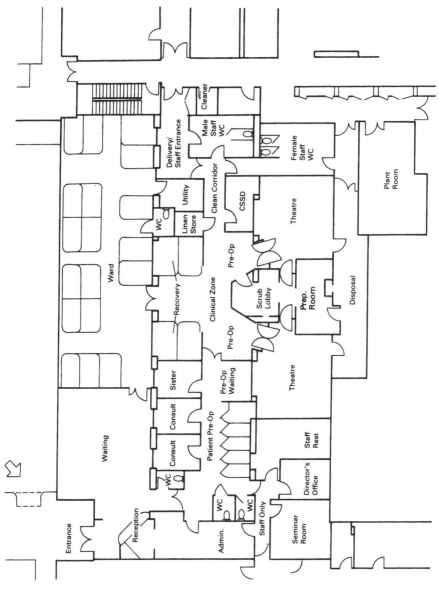

Fig. 1.1 A typical day surgery unit plan (adapted with permission from Addenbrooke's NHS Trust).

and (where appropriate) when to shave the operation site. It should be noted at pre-assessment whether a patient is able to comply with these requirements as the elderly and infirm often find it difficult, in which case arrangements must be made for nursing staff to perform these tasks on admission day. Facilities should also be available for patients and staff to shower and change.

The activity in any day unit is normally high, with a constant throughput and high turnover of patients and accompanying relatives. The traffic flow should be from one area to another without any cross flows or backtracking. Special attention must be paid to the cleanliness of the ward area and at which times of the day hoovering and damp dusting are to be carried out. Domestic staff are important members of the day surgery team and should be included in the drawing up of policies and procedures which affect their work.

As to causes of infection, we must remember that it is people and not clothes that are the major source, due to shedding of microorganisms from the hair, skin and perineum. Theatre staff should always cover hair, and high filtration masks should be worn by all staff at all times in the theatre area. Masks and (where appropriate) aprons should also be worn by the endoscopy staff. Goggles and face shields should be worn where appropriate and, most importantly, if there is to be any splashing or use of lasers.

Many patients find that the theatre environment is both frightening and intimidating but fortunately 'patient comfort devices', such as personal stereos and toys for children, have been shown not to pose any major infection risk and should be allowed.

Large pieces of equipment, such as laser devices and resuscitation trolleys, should always be covered when not in use. Sterile items should be stored off the floor and at a level which avoids their being splashed by mops when cleaning or touched repeatedly by hand. Reprocessing and reuse of disposables remains controversial although these practices are not uncommon. Policies for such methods must be in place and carefully evaluated. Fixed equipment, such as lights, shelves and blinds should be cleaned on a regular basis at a time when the theatre is not in use. This also applies to the air handling system.

Infection control continues to evolve and flexibility is required in the implementation and progress of any infection control programme. It requires all staff to be vigilant and to pay attention to detail. Above all it involves a great deal of common sense.

Patient and staff safety

To date, the mortality reported in association with day surgery is very low and the call to be prepared for a disaster needs constant reinforcement. The morbidity to be most feared involves the respiratory and circulatory systems and is rare in day care patients, and mainly determined by the pre-existing disease. Safety therefore commences with the day unit assessment of the appropriate patients for day care, which is fortified by good patient information and communication. The day care team must be aware of and committed to policies of safety just as rigorous as those which apply to patients within the hospital. Routine rehearsals should ensure every staff member knows how to respond to an emergency. Subjects range from standard cardio–pulmonary resuscitation to locating the regime and the drugs for malignant hyperthermia treatment. Advances in both medical and surgical technology bring new risks, and these can extend day surgery to the less fit, requiring even more emphasis on the safety programme.

Health and safety regulations apply to all day care staff just as to those within hospital. It is important to remember that many of the day care staff may be part-time or juniors, who may have a less complete understanding of a unit's rules and the reasons for them, but must still be able to carry them out. Body fluids and specimens are potentially dangerous and must be handled with particular care. Fire and electrical hazards exist so due precautions are called for together with knowledge of the action required in the event of an incident.

Medical legal questions

The legal standards required of staff are the same whether a patient is an in-patient or has day care. Additional risks with day care are created by the provision of pre-assessment, as the patient is seen by fewer people after referral by a GP – usually just a consultant in out-patients and the pre-assessment nurse. There are not the extensive checks on arrival for surgery that occur on in-patient admittance. The concentration of procedures within a limited time and the fact that aftercare does not have continuous on-site expert attention also create risk. Reduced contact with patients can lessen the rapport which can be so important in handling real or imagined grievances and the conduct of nurses, who have the greatest amount of contact with day care patients, is crucial. The majority of patients are fit and undergo simpler operations with less risk, which means that the rare incident may therefore be considered more disastrous. With the construction of units away from the hospital infrastructure, the organisation of any unit, rather than its location, should define the type of work which can be undertaken without serious medico–legal risk. In a free-standing unit special staffing arrangements may be needed – for example in the United States, a doctor with resuscitation skills is required on site until all patients leave.

Because of the managerial and directional work which nurses may take on in day surgery, it may be necessary to extend clinical insurance, provided by a protection society, to these other functions. Certainly advice should be sought on this aspect of legal cover. Health service marketing may give the public unreal expectations, therefore such promotions should be checked by clinicians. As always, records are vital in any legal matter and need always to be conscientiously and meticulously kept even under the pressure of the rapid processing of patients. Any corrections on records must be left readable and explained; always cross out and do not erase. Everyone must abide by the policies in force, and if they are in need of change it must be done quickly, as

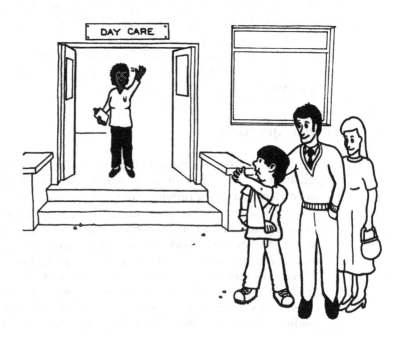

an intention without subsequent action may be considered legally culpable.

Insisting that patients have day surgery against their wishes is as legally indefensible as undertaking a treatment to which they have not agreed. Patients who do not appear, do not read information or leave against advice must be treated with cool circumspection so they do not harass staff and create medical legal perils. In the event of a catastrophic death in day surgery, the structured in-patient procedure should be carried out meticulously with compassion and thus lessen the likelihood of subsequent litigation.

Key messages

(1) For a large number of patients, surgical and medical care without admission to hospital is clinically and socially good.
(2) Day care departments need to be specially designed, and where there is sufficient demand, they should be self-sufficient.
(3) Day care saves on hotel, hospital, routine and nursing costs but is an intense service and is not cheap.
(4) Safety arrangements for day care must be organised, known and understood by all staff and patients, and reviewed regularly.

References and further reading

Association of Anaesthetists of Great Britain and Ireland *Day Case Surgery: The Anaesthetist's Role in Promoting High Quality Care*, Association of Anaesthetists, London, 1994.

Audit Commission *A Short Cut to Better Services – Day Surgery in England and Wales*, HMSO, London, 1990.

Audit Commission *Measuring Quality: The Patients' View of Day Surgery*, HMSO, London, 1991.

Audit Commission *All in a Day's Work – Summary of an Audit of Day Surgery in England and Wales: An Occasional Paper of the Audit Commission*, HMSO, London, 1992.

Audit Commission *Lying in Wait – The Use of Medical Beds in Acute Hospitals*, HMSO, London, 1992.

Cohen, D. and Dillon, J.B. 'Anesthesia for out-patient surgery', *Journal of the American Medical Association*, 196 (1966), 987.

Ford, J.L. and Reed, W.A. 'The surgicentre – an innovation in the delivery and cost of medical care', *Arizona Medicine*, 26 (1969), 801.

Jacobs, P., Nichols, D. and Dubitz, T. *Comparative Costs of Substitutable Services: In-Patient and Day Surgery Episodes of Care*, University of Ottawa, Canada, 1994.

National Health Building Note no. 52 *Part 1 – Day Surgery Unit. Part 2 – Endoscopy Unit. Part 3 – Medical Investigation and Treatment Unit*, HMSO, London, 1994.

National Health Service Management Executive *Day Surgery Report and Tool Kit – Report by the Day Surgery Task Force*, Health Publications Unit, Heywood, 1993.

Nicoll, J.H. 'A surgery of infancy', *British Medical Journal*, 2 (1909), 753.

Partridge, A.D., Brennan, M.F. and Gray, N.H. *Day Surgery – Making it Happen: A Study Conducted by the NHS Management Executive Value-for-Money Unit*, HMSO, London, 1991.

The Royal College of Surgeons of England *Commission on the Provision of Surgical Services. Guidelines for Day Case Surgery*, Royal College of Surgeons, London, 1985.

The Royal College of Surgeons of England *Guidelines for Day Case Surgery* (revised edition), Royal College of Surgeons, London, 1992.

Thornes, R. *Just for the Day: Children Admitted to Hospital for Day Treatment*, NAWCH Ltd, London, 1991.

Waters, R.M. 'The downtown anesthesia clinic', *American Journal of Surgery*, 33 (1919), 71.

Chapter 2

Day Surgery Management and Organisation

Sarah Penn

Introduction

One of the key factors for a successful day surgery unit is competent management, as was highlighted in the reports on day surgery from the Audit Commission and the Value-for-Money Unit of the National Health Service Executive. The principles of management are to plan, direct, organise and control the activities of employees to achieve or exceed objectives. Establishing the workload, financial planning, clear lines of responsibility and personnel management are the components of any managerial technique.

Management structure

Day-to-day management and organisation of a day surgery unit is best performed by a nurse. This is because the nurse processes a patient through the whole undertaking and can unite the clinical and logistic aspects of this work. Managing a day surgery unit is a challenging task that requires good communication skills, marketing and financial expertise and effective organisational competence which, when the job is performed well, will lead to a high level of job satisfaction. It is a multifaceted role which balances the needs of patients, nursing, medical and ancillary staff, management, purchasers and the community all at the same time.

A clinical director of day surgery should also be appointed. This is usually a surgeon or anaesthetist who is enthusiastic about day surgery and will have an active role in the unit. The clinical director and manager must work closely together, measuring activity with contracts, overseeing the expenditure and marketing, writing business plans, maintaining quality initiatives and overseeing educational programmes. At Addenbrooke's Hospital day surgery unit a regular fortnightly meeting of the senior staff takes place and a monthly meeting is held which involves all the unit staff.

A day surgery unit users' committee should be established, preferably at the planning stage of any new unit. This committee should include representation from the surgeons, anaesthetists, management and nursing staff, and it is appropriate that the clinical director chairs these meetings on a two- or three-monthly basis. The committee's function is to agree strategies and to update policies, and it provides a multidisciplinary forum to enhance communication channels. With a comprehensive quality assurance system in place (see Chapter 10), the committee may use its results to improve the unit utilisation as well as to improve the quality of the service.

As hospitals move towards the target of 70% of elective surgery being performed on a day care basis, many day units provide a large enough service to function independently of other areas within the hospital structure. In this case overall responsibility for the budget should be held by the clinical director and the manager. Depending on the size of the hospital it may be appropriate for the clinical director to have a position on the Trust Board. The manager must have an established line of responsibility, for instance to the director of nursing services or, through other management channels, to the chief executive or their deputy.

It is vital that the day care unit has an updated operational policy and this document should have the support of the day users' committee. It should enable managers to perform their job secure in the knowledge that there is a strict framework which all personnel ought to abide by. The operational policy document requires updating annually to incorporate the introduction of new surgical and anaesthetic techniques and the changes in policies which may result from audit, research findings and nursing development. The guidelines for content of an operational policy are as follows:

(1) Definition of day surgery.
(2) Unit philosophy and objectives.
(3) Accommodation and facilities:
        plans, opening hours, session times.
(4) Management structure:
        organisational chart, meetings.

(5)   Pre-admission policies:
      patient selection, anaesthetic criteria, social criteria, pre-
      operative assessment.
(6)   Booking of patients:
      allocation of sessions, case mix.
(7)   Protocols:
      reception, pre-operative, preparation, operating theatre,
      recovery, ward areas.
(8)   Discharge and aftercare:
      procedures, patient information, liaison with general
      practitioners and community services, transfer of
      patients unfit for discharge.
(9)   Policies for special groups, such as paediatrics.
(10) Quality assurance programme.
(11) Health and safety measures:
      fire drill, major incident plan.
(12) Managerial issues:
      contracts, staffing levels, job descriptions, finances.
(13) Examples of paperwork:
      care plans, patient information.
(14) A list of support services provided.

Establishment and skill mix

The aim of the manager is to use human resources both efficiently
and effectively. For many years the human resource structure in
the NHS has been far too rigid and an opportunity to review the
skill mix should be welcomed. It is to the manager's advantage to
review establishment levels and skill mix periodically as this will
provide a much stronger case when studied by senior management and external agencies. The results can be included in the
business plan to provide information on future service planning.

Many day surgery units are ahead of the field in this area as
multiskilling has already been introduced. The preferred option
for day units is to be in integrated, self-contained facilities, and
this has made the introduction of multiskilling beneficial for
economic reasons and in terms of job satisfaction. If the day unit is
separate, with patients being operated upon in the main theatre
complex, the same approach to assessing the required establishment and skill mix should be undertaken.

The purpose of a skill mix review is to identify the ideal skill
mix for future staffing levels and to give an opportunity to

question previous patterns of staff utilisation. A suggested framework for achieving this exercise is demonstrated in the list below.

(1) Specify the purpose and the objectives of the unit.

(2) List:
  • description of the facilities/areas to be staffed;
  • different client groups; and
  • support services.
    (Include guidelines for staffing levels from professional bodies, such as the National Association of Theatre Nurses and British Society of Gastroenterologists – staffing endoscopy units.)

(3) For each session list:
  • tasks and grade of staff required to perform them; and
  • average time taken to perform task, for instance 20 minutes for pre-admission patient assessment.
    (Include staff required to manage the unit, administrative and clerical tasks, and basic tasks that require supervision by a trained member of staff.)

  Identify the usual number of students in the unit.

(4) Validate the data collected, and review the tasks and grade required by discussion.

(5) Specify the minimum level of cover and skill mix for each session. Use this data to calculate weekly cover and Whole Time Equivalents and add percentage for annual leave/ sickness/study leave according to hospital policy.

  Measure this against current establishment.

(6) Review the current job descriptions.

The manager should analyse new developments and the staffing requirements as they occur. Funding for any necessary increase should be sought before implementing the required changes, or the workload will expand before new personnel are taken on, causing staff stress and a lowering of morale.

It is sometimes surprising how an improvement to the service can make untold demands on the staff. At Addenbrooke's Hospital day surgery unit telephoning the patients the day after surgery was perceived as a major quality initiative. An audit was carried out to assess the benefits of implementing the telephone calls using a patient questionnaire, which proved the perception right. When the calls were timed, it was discovered that an experienced qualified nurse took an average of three minutes per call, and for the number of required calls it took five hours of nursing time per week (costed at mid E grade). Senior management is far more likely to fund such initiatives when the data is presented to them in a comprehensive way before a service is implemented.

Personnel management

It is impossible to achieve a smooth running service which maintains high quality and safe patient care without looking after the staff. Personnel management is a major element of the manager's role. It includes:

- recruitment
- staff development
- appraisal
- discipline.

Recruitment

Paul Windolf, writing in *Introducing Management*, says:

'Recruitment and selection may be used deliberately to stabilize the status quo of an organization or, alternatively, to bring about innovation and social change.'

Selecting the right member of staff to join the team needs careful consideration and there is no easy formula to ensure the correct decision is made. One of the most important elements required by the nursing staff is the ability to establish an immediate rapport with the large number of people who pass through a busy day surgery unit.

Before considering the applicants it is helpful to make a list of the key elements that you require so that you have a consistent basis on which to measure their qualities. There are almost certainly specific skills which are essential for the particular post that is to be filled, especially in a unit where multiskilling is practised; for example it may be necessary to insist on theatre skills or, on the other hand, it might be possible to acquire those skills at a later stage as part of an educational programme. As day surgery expands and more day surgery courses are completed, it will become easier to find nurses prepared for or with experience in the speciality. Below is a list of characteristics which should be looked for in any day surgery nurse:

- good communication skills
- a caring attitude
- ability to organise and prioritise
- a team player
- ability to cope with fast throughput of patients
- enthusiasm and motivation
- self confidence
- attention to detail
- adaptability.

Staff development

The manager must take on the responsibility of encouraging staff development. Leading by example is a good way to motivate the staff and this can be achieved by becoming involved in professional organisations such as the British Association of Day Surgery, the National Association of Theatre Nurses or the Royal College of Nursing Specialist Group of Day Surgery Nurses. The list is expansive if one considers the speciality client groups that are involved in day surgery, such as paediatrics, ophthalmics, orthopaedics and endoscopy. The staff must also be encouraged to participate in activities outside their own unit, as much may be learned from their peers in other areas of health care.

Day surgery offers scope for a multitude of skills and areas of interest. The specific educational courses for day surgery nurses and other training programmes are described in Chapter 3. Through implementing a variety of courses a workforce that is multiskilled but with a wide range of special interests and expertise can be achieved. Objective setting and an annual performance appraisal system are essential to provide a formal guarantee that there is continuous professional growth because it is easy to overlook some members of staff if there are a few ambitious nurses who regularly appropriate study leave.

Objective setting

Staff should be encouraged to set their own objectives before discussing them with the manager. These objectives should reflect educational issues, expansion of roles and personal areas of interest that, in turn, will benefit the unit. Timescales for attaining these objectives should be realistic and objective setting ought to be an ongoing process through the year. Objectives should be:

(1)   Definable – expressed in a meaningful way.
(2)   Attainable – challenging enough to stretch the individual, but not unrealistic.
(3)   Specific – success criteria must be defined by the appraiser.
(4)   Relevant – relate to the work of the individual.
(5)   Measurable – specify either quantity (how much) or quality (how well).
(6)   Agreed jointly – this ensures a two-way commitment.
(7)   Summarised and incorporated into an action plan.

Performance review

Individual performance review is a system that helps each job holder to:

(1)   Be clear about what job performance is expected of him/her.
(2)   Identify short- and long-term goals.
(3)   Receive feedback from the manager.
(4)   Understand how his/her own job ties in with and affects the work of others.

Performance review offers a formal opportunity to discuss an individual's ambitions and concerns in a non-threatening way. This does not mean, however, that it is the only time these discussions should take place. Staff should feel that they are able to approach the manager or appraiser at any mutually convenient time, whenever they have a concern or want to discuss their professional development. It is helpful if the manager has kept notes in each staff member's records during the year so that discussions, particular achievements and situations dealt with can be reviewed during the formal appraisal. The purpose of performance review is to:

(1)   Agree standards; managers and staff should have a common understanding of the expected level of performance and what a successful outcome might be.
(2)   Review past performance and progress.

(3) Examine (where appropriate) the staff member's management style.
(4) Establish objectives over a defined period.
(5) Provide a forum for discussion; performance appraisal is an exercise in two-way communication.
(6) Identify training required for individuals to meet their objectives and development needs.
(7) Discuss the staff member's potential and future career aspirations/prospects.
(8) Motivate the staff member and enhance their personal interest in the job.
(9) Strengthen the departmental team in terms of personal relationships, thus hopefully reducing tension and anxiety.

It must be remembered that performance review is not an alternative to day-to-day monitoring of an individual's performance and ongoing feedback. It must also not be used as an annual purge, an exercise in bureaucracy or a time for character assassination.

Prior to performing an appraisal ensure that individuals know and understand the purpose of the discussions and give them time to prepare. Fix a date and time in advance for each appraisal

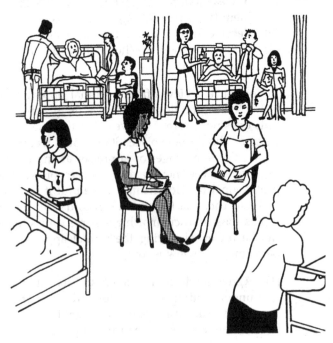

and do not cancel at the last minute as this will leave the individual feeling frustrated, anxious and undervalued.

Feedback should be constructive rather than destructive and give the individual an opportunity to change. Key points in giving feedback are:

(1) Start with the positive.
(2) Be specific in praise and criticism.
(3) Focus on behaviour that can be changed – appraise performance not personality.
(4) Be descriptive rather than evaluative.
(5) Ask questions rather than make statements – staff members can then take responsibility for reaching their own conclusions.
(6) Limit negative feedback – give a priority order to issues and concentrate on the most important ones.

A constructive performance review system will benefit individuals, the manager and the department as a whole. The individual should come away from the interview feeling that the most has been made of the opportunity to talk freely about the job.

Discipline

The hospital human resource department will have policies on disciplinary issues ranging from the initial identification of a problem to dismissal, and these should be followed. The notes made by the manager which are mentioned in the section on performance review, notes of any counselling sessions and proof of offered guidance will be valuable in any disciplinary action.

Establishing the workload

An increase in day case treatment as an alternative to in-patient care is a principal national objective. To establish the workload, many factors have to be taken into consideration and this will involve external agencies (purchasers, including general practice (GP) fundholders, Regional Health Authority and District Health Authority planners and contract staff, public health staff, Community Health Councils and general practitioners (GPs)) as well as the hospital or provider unit staff. Those involved on the provider unit side will be general managers, business managers, the director and manager of the day surgery unit, and clinicians. Although this is a complicated process, it is easier in day surgery than in other areas of health care as only elective surgery is being planned. Workload assessment is a perpetual task.

The remainder of this chapter will focus on planning the workload at the clinical director and manager level. This involves marketing, writing business plans and dealing with the contracting agreements, none of which can be done without a knowledge of the hospital's objectives and capital plans.

Marketing

One of the most common complaints made by day surgery nurses is that the rest of the hospital thinks they work in the 'lump and bump clinic' and that the amount and complexity of the surgery performed is not appreciated. In these circumstances, the day surgery nurses themselves are seriously to blame because they should take on more of the responsibility for raising the profile of modern day surgery. Day surgery nursing is at the forefront of many of the changes in nursing practice and has extended the boundaries of conventional patient care. On many issues, such as pre-admission assessment and patient discharge, the nurses on hospital surgical wards can learn from day surgery research. If other departments within the provider unit are not aware of day surgery developments and quality issues, how can we expect the purchasers, GPs, practice and community health care workers to know?

Raising the profile of day surgery within any hospital is not a difficult exercise and can be done by all members of staff by:

- attending meetings other than specific day surgery meetings, such as nurse policy groups
- teaching within the unit
- volunteering to talk to the local college of nursing about day surgery on various courses
- establishing close links with the specialities that use the unit, for instance the paediatric unit or the ophthalmic wards
- joining related professional organisations like the National Association of Theatre Nurses.

Raising the profile outside the hospital requires more effort but is important in the purchasing scenario. Purchasers of health care and GPs need to know what their local day surgery unit has to offer in terms of the type of procedures performed and, importantly, the quality care which their patients will receive. It is often by demand from those buying health care services that the impetus for an increase in day surgery will be made.

Contact should be made by inviting purchasers, GPs, practice nurses, community nurses and the Community Health Council into the unit on a series of open evenings. A tour of the facilities, an explanation of how a patient is treated from pre-admission to discharge, audit results and examples of patient information leaflets can be presented. A model patient may be asked to come along to relate their experience of day surgery in the unit.

Another means of contact is to visit GPs' surgeries to talk to the staff about day surgery, or to attend one of their meetings. Day unit staff may volunteer to speak at GPs' training sessions or at practice nurse meetings. Furthermore, when patient information leaflets are produced or updated, copies should be sent to the local GP surgeries so they are aware of the instructions being given to their patients. At the same time, it is possible to ask GPs for their opinion of the advice given to patients in the leaflets.

It helps to keep in touch with other local provider units. It makes economic sense to work together in deciding which procedures to perform and where, rather than to remain in competition. For example, ophthalmic surgery is an expensive speciality to establish so it is essential to know if there is enough work for two units that are close together. If not, one unit could offer ophthalmic surgery while the other offers another speciality that is in demand.

Business plans

A business plan for day surgery needs to be developed in conjunction with the surgical divisions of the hospital. It should inform senior management of the requirements to expand the day surgery service, both in volume and quality terms, and should give an idea of the capital outlay needed. The impact of day surgery expansion on in-patient services should be taken into account. The business plan will be used in helping with the contracting arrangements for elective surgery in the year ahead. The following are key elements of a day surgery business plan:

- a summary of the present arrangements for day surgery
- an assessment of the future demand

- various options for meeting the future demand
- proposals for delivering a day surgery strategy.

Present arrangements for day surgery

These should include:

(a) Day surgery facilities – current locations of day surgery activity; number of beds and available theatre sessions; available equipment for specific procedures; and provision for specific specialities such as paediatrics or endoscopy.

(b) Management issues – management responsibility; administrative policies (e.g. pre-admission assessment of patients); and establishment levels including nursing, administrative personnel and consultant staff who perform day surgery.

(c) Statistics – type and current amount of day surgery performed by speciality and procedure.

(d) Community liaison – GPs' referral methods; use of community or practice nurses.

Future demand for day surgery services

(a) Requests from clinicians for their appraisal of extra throughput or new procedures.

(b) Levels of day surgery requested by purchasers, by speciality and procedure; purchasers' quality specifications.

(c) External agencies' views, such as results of GPs' satisfaction surveys or discussions with Community Health Council; procedures being undertaken in primary health care units; and results of patient satisfaction surveys highlighting deficiencies.

(d) Other provider units – current position against local and regional best practice.

(e) Summary of the required increase in day surgery – current numbers and procedures performed against purchasers' targets; and broad outline of implications of increase, for instance theatre capacity or equipment required.

Options for meeting the future demand

(a) Detailed analysis of increasing day surgery by speciality – theatre sessions required; number of beds; impact on sur-

geon and anaesthetist workload; equipment requirements; and training needs.
(b) List the various options available for meeting the demand with costs and benefits (include limitations, such as surgeons who choose not to perform certain procedures on a day case basis).

Proposals for delivering a day surgery strategy

This is the section of the document that details the development of the service and should include:

(a) A summary of the preferred option for increasing the service with reasons for this choice.
(b) Reference to and future requirements of – facilities, equipment, staffing levels, educational needs, information systems.
(c) Quality assurance measures.
(d) Marketing strategies.

Contracts

A contract is a business agreement between two parties for supplying goods or performing work at a specified price. In the day surgery unit this involves the purchasers and the providers agreeing which procedures will be undertaken, the volume and the price. The purchasers will look at all of the provider units within their locality in terms of the service offered, the costs and the quality of patient care. Quality issues are of paramount importance and the purchasers will not necessarily choose the cheapest option. They want the best care possible while maintaining value for money, and day surgery managers must be aware of the quality issues that will interest purchasers. They must collect the data to substantiate claims that a high quality service is being offered and this subject is dealt with in Chapter 10.

It is important to establish realistic contracts that can be met within the specified time limit, otherwise the service will suffer. If the contracts are too high and the work is not achieved there are financial penalties imposed by the purchasers. If they are too small, the work may be completed after nine months instead of twelve, and then the facilities may have to be used for another purpose or the staff relocated elsewhere, which disbands the team spirit.

In an established day unit the basis of estimating the workload is to take the average number of patients per session for each consultant. This figure is then multiplied by the number of sessions that each consultant will perform over the year, remembering to deduct some time for annual and study leave and bank holidays. Some consultants have senior registrars that can perform the work in their absence but others will have to cancel their lists if they are unavailable. A total number of cases per speciality can then be deduced. Adjustments to the timetable may be required if the number of sessions available for each speciality are inadequate to achieve the required number of cases specified during the contract negotiations. This task requires discussions with the consultants involved and with other departments in the hospital, for example theatres and out-patient departments, as an alteration to the timetable in the day unit may impact on their schedules.

The manager should monitor throughput of the unit by speciality on a regular basis. These data will provide the information on how closely the agreed contracts are being achieved and the day unit timetable may need adjusting during the year if any speciality is under- or over-performing, so that at the end of the year agreed targets are met.

Key messages

(1) Day surgery management requires full team cooperation and communication.

(2) The ideal day surgery nurse is multiskilled and patient orientated.

(3) Assessing staff performance should be seen as a positive manoeuvre for the individual and the service.

(4) Marketing and business planning are the basis of contract completion in the new health service.

References and further reading

Audit Commission *A Short Cut to Better Services – Day Surgery in England and Wales*, HMSO, London, 1990.

Bevan, P.G. *The Management and Utilisation of Operating Departments. A Study Conducted by the NHS Management Executive Value-for-Money Unit*, HMSO, London, 1989.

Bradshaw, E.G. and Davenport H.T. *Day Care – Surgery, Anaesthesia and Management*, Edward Arnold, London, 1989.

Burden, N. *Ambulatory Surgical Nursing*, W.B. Saunders, London, 1993.

Lawrence, P. and Elliott, K. *Introducing Management*, Penguin Business, London, 1985.

National Health Service Management Executive *Day Surgery Report and Tool Kit – Report by the Day Surgery Task Force*, Health Publications Unit, Heywood, 1993.

Ogg, T.W., Heath, P. and Brownlie, G. 'A case for the expansion of day surgery', *Health Trends*, 21: 4 (1989), 114–17.

Ogg, T.W. and Watson, B.J. *Anaesthesia Rounds – Aspects of Day Surgery and Anaesthesia: A Multidisciplinary Approach*, Zeneca Pharmaceuticals, Medicine Group Education Ltd, Abingdon, 1995.

Partridge, A.D., Brennan, M.F. and Gray, N.H. *Day Surgery – Making it Happen: A Study Conducted by the NHS Management Executive Value-for-Money Unit*, HMSO, London, 1991.

The Royal College of Surgeons of England *Guidelines for Day Case Surgery* (revised edition), Royal College of Surgeons, London, 1992.

Thornes, R. *Just for the Day: Children Admitted to Hospital for Day Treatment*, NAWCH Ltd, London, 1991.

Chapter 3
Education in Day Surgery

Sarah Penn

Introduction

There is a need for specialist training and education in the rapidly expanding field of day surgery for all members of the team involved. It is only through education and research that day surgery will flourish and continue to provide the quality specialist care to which all patients are entitled. The Royal College of Surgeons, the Audit Commission and the NHS Management Executive have all acknowledged the training needs of surgeons, anaesthetists and nurses. Specialist higher award courses in day surgery for nurses started in 1992, as the English National Board (ENB) recognised its different educational needs from the available surgical nursing courses.

This chapter addresses orientation programmes for new members of staff in day surgery, continuing education opportunities for day surgery nurses and specific day surgery or perioperative and day care nursing courses. A section outlining the educational requirements of other day unit staff is included.

It is both efficient and economical to employ nursing staff who are competent to work in any area of the day surgery unit. With the nurses rotating through the various areas of an integrated day surgery facility a sense of teamwork is generated and this is essential for the smooth running of the service. Nurses appreciate the concept of total patient care in its true sense because they are involved in patient education and counselling as well as the critical care aspect of the theatre environment. There is a limited variety of procedures in day care, but those few must be performed frequently so nurses appreciate a rotation which prevents the boredom of routine. To take on the many aspects of nurse rotation the nurses should be trained to a high level and an experienced day surgery nurse ought to be capable of the following:

- communicating with and educating the patients and their carers
- assessing and pre-operatively screening patients following agreed medical and social guidelines
- assisting the surgeon, 'circulating' and helping the anaesthetist
- recovering unconscious patients
- discharging patients safely with the correct information
- maintaining a high level of total patient care.

In addition to these subjects they should be proficient in:

- management
- teaching
- computing
- cooperating with all the day care team.

While experienced day surgery nurses should be skilled in all these tasks they may also be experts in specific areas such as paediatrics, ophthalmics or patient information. These experts provide a resource for all members of staff and the patients benefit from being cared for in an environment with highly skilled practitioners.

Orientation programmes

Orientation programmes for new members of staff should be specifically devised to take into consideration their previous knowledge and experience, their strengths and weaknesses, and thus their specific training needs. The length of time needed for orientation will vary considerably depending on how much of the new staff members' previous experience is relevant to day care.

A preceptor or key worker should be allocated to oversee the new members of staff orientation programme. The preceptor should be chosen carefully and should take on the role willingly. Good teaching and communication skills are required for the preceptorship role as well as sound clinical experience. The teacher and student should work closely together to establish a rapport and to ensure that the newcomers' learning objectives are met.

The day surgery unit should produce an implicit basic programme for the orientation of any new member of staff. This should include:

(1) The operational policy with specific emphasis on:
 • the unit philosophy
 • management structure
 • quality assurance programme.
(2) Both the hospital and the unit policies and procedures.
(3) Fire drill.
(4) Resuscitation training.
(5) The Patient's Charter.
(6) The United Kingdom Central Council for Nursing, Midwifery and Health Visiting (UKCC) Code of Conduct.
(7) A suggested reading list of relevant day surgery documents, books and papers.

Most hospitals provide an orientation programme for new employees which includes some of these global training requirements and attendance at these courses should be compulsory.

A tour of the hospital is usually included in the hospital's induction programme. However, specific visits to departments and especially meetings with those who work closely with the day surgery unit should be organised, for instance the theatre sterile supplies unit, physiotherapy department and out-patient clinics.

The specific training needs of an individual may require experience being gained outside the day surgery unit. For example, a trained theatre nurse may never have worked in a particular speciality such as ophthalmics and may benefit from a period of time spent in that speciality's in-patient area. A nurse with no recovery experience should gain experience and be deemed competent in an in-patient environment before recovering patients unsupervised in day surgery. Specific elements of individual orientation programmes can include:

• pre-operative assessment
• patient selection criteria
• patient education and health promotion
• critical care training including theatre, anaesthetic and recovery elements
• patient discharge policies
• management and organisational issues
• endoscopy training.

Every new member of staff should initially be supervised and assessed as being competent before embarking on any unsupervised practice in day care.

Further education

There are many opportunities within day surgery for continuing education and professional development. As most surgical specialities now do day surgery the nursing staff can gain experience and further their education in many directions, thus giving them an opportunity to shape their own career in a variety of ways.

The educational system in nursing has changed dramatically over the past few years and has become far more flexible. In day surgery this has helped managers develop teams of highly trained personnel, and to develop a diverse workforce by encouraging expertise in specific areas of patient care. The most important change is the modularisation of post-basic courses which enables practitioners to complete all the modules of specific courses to obtain ENB specialist certificates or to undertake appropriate individual modules that will meet their own learning needs. As modules are credit rated, nurses are able to study them as individual courses, as part of the BSc (Hons) Professional Nursing Practice or within the ENB requirements of the Higher Award Scheme. There is also a flexibility in the time span in which modules may be completed, which is beneficial for both individual students and for managers who can plan study leave accordingly.

A few of the modules are also accessible to other health care workers, for example operating department practitioners, and advice should be sought from the individual colleges of education.

Nurses who take a selection of the courses listed below will enhance their professional development and be an asset to any day surgery unit:

- teaching and assessment courses, e.g. ENB 998, City & Guilds 730, work-based assessors courses
- theatre and anaesthetic nurse courses, e.g. ENB 183, 925 or 776
- recovery nurse courses
- surgical nursing courses, e.g. ENB A25
- professional knowledge and research
- health promotion

- family planning
- paediatric nursing
- specialist certificates, e.g. ophthalmic, orthopaedic, endo-scopy nursing
- counselling
- alternative therapy courses, e.g. massage
- management courses
- community nursing
- perioperative and day care nursing, e.g. ENB A21, N33.

Specialist day surgery courses

Although the expansion of day surgery in the UK was initially slow, in recent years it has developed rapidly. New technology has altered surgical practice and led to improved anaesthetic agents and pain relief techniques, while economic considerations and the realisation of the importance of quality issues have also played their part in the expansion of day surgery and the change in delivery of patient care. Nurses in the day care setting need continuing educational opportunities to keep abreast of these changes and courses are also necessary to provide a sound knowledge base for nurses who staff the new day surgery units that are rapidly being provided. The concept of specialist day surgery courses evolved from this need.

There are two English National Board courses:

- ENB A21 – Perioperative and Day Care Nursing Practice
- ENB N33 – A Short Course in Perioperative and Day Care Nursing Practice.

These courses have been updated and modularised along with the recent changes in the educational system and the title of the courses may vary slightly. Nurses who complete the shorter ENB N33 course have the opportunity to APEL (Accreditation of Prior Experiential Learning) into the longer ENB A21 course at a later date. In most cases, the ENB A21 has common core modules, such as professional studies and research, that support other courses, as well as specialist modules specific to perioperative day care. Both courses consist of both theory and practice and include elements of the following subjects:

- nursing practice and the delivery of care

- professional studies, such as research, teaching, management and organisation, ethics, and legal professional accountability
- health promotion
- biological sciences, for instance applied anatomy, microbiology and pharmacology
- psychology and sociology which apply to the specialist setting of day surgery.

Pre-registration students

Day surgery offers a conducive environment for pre-registration students to learn about surgical patient care. The close links between the community and the hospital setting make it an ideal place to learn about total patient care.

Many routine surgical cases have now been moved from the inpatient wards to the day surgery unit and unless day surgery is included in pre-registration courses, students will miss a vital element of their training. This is true for students undertaking both the adult and the paediatric branches of nurse training, as well as medical students and operating department practitioners.

The trained day surgery nurses should be prepared to take on this teaching role, to help students set and achieve their learning aims. Having students in the day unit will also help to encourage staff recruitment, as many will appreciate gaining experience in a wide range of work.

Educational audit

In order to offer a learning environment for students, units will be obliged to undergo an educational audit to satisfy the colleges that their standard of practice is high enough for teaching strategies. Educational audits should be looked on in a positive way as they help to ensure that trained staff are kept up to date with new nursing theories, that teaching resources are available and that research is fostered.

Educational audits are normally carried out annually by the college to which students are attached. The unit is required to complete a document of standards, stating that it can meet certain criteria. Evidence of ongoing professional development will be asked for, as well as establishment levels and the qualifications of the permanent staff. Orientation packs for students, educational resource information and paperwork, such as care plans, will need to be seen. A surveyor, usually a tutor from the college, will then visit the unit to discuss the document and to look for evidence that the criteria have been fulfilled. All members of the day surgery unit should be involved in this process, as it is the unit that is being audited, not the manager or any particular member of staff.

In areas where any students are placed, there should be a link tutor who can liaise between the college and the unit. This tutor can play an active role in the unit by being available to help all members of staff. For example, when interviewing candidates for a vacant post, the link tutor can be asked to be an external advisor. Often this will provide someone with an insight into the requirements of the unit, but with perhaps a wider view than the day unit staff. An enthusiastic link tutor may also be prepared to help trained members of staff with their own professional development or perhaps to advise them on their personal portfolios. Trained members of staff who are acting as preceptors or key workers for students need support, and this ought to be a major part of the link tutor's role.

The process of completing educational audits is much smoother and less threatening when there is a regular input from the college through an active link tutor. As with all audits, if higher standards are aimed for, patient care will benefit. After all, audit is about measuring how far you are from where you want to be and then changing practice accordingly in order to achieve those higher standards.

UKCC PREP (Post-Registration Education and Practice) (1994)

The educational variety and flexibility which day surgery offers means there are numerous ways of ensuring that all staff can adhere to the PREP recommendations. Study days are numerous, both in the day surgery field and in related specialities, for example endoscopy or paediatrics. Managers will come to appreciate the enthusiastic nurse who is willing to forego a day off in order to gain personal professional development.

Due to the fact that the work in a day surgery unit is largely elective, many units may close or reduce their workload substantially so that the staff can attend relevant conferences, such as the British Association of Day Surgery Annual General and Scientific Meetings. These meetings not only address PREP but develop a network of interested people who will help to improve the delivery of patient care.

In-house teaching sessions

Time should be allocated regularly for teaching and audit within any day care unit. Medical staff are all obliged to have clinical audit sessions and, within the day unit, interdisciplinary teaching should be inherent. In many units the anaesthetists have an audit afternoon on a monthly basis, and managers of day units ought to use these sessions for teaching within the unit rather than filling the time with lists of local anaesthetic cases. Alternatively perhaps an hour at the end of the day can be utilised. All staff should attend and the following subjects can be discussed:

- audits
- resuscitation updates
- fire drill
- new nursing issues
- speciality topics, such as paediatrics/ophthalmics
- feedback from nurses who have attended courses/seminars/conferences.

The list is wide-ranging, but these teaching sessions offer an opportunity for all staff to participate and to take on teaching roles. Day surgery nurses have an advantage over most other nurses in that, due to the planned, elective nature of their work, it should be possible to plan teaching sessions.

Other personnel

All day surgery staff require specialist training, and managers should remember this when planning study leave and educational budgets.

Day surgery should be a specialist aspect of the operating department practitioners training course if they are employed within day units. An operating department practitioner who is competent in a cardiac theatre may not be ideal in a day surgery unit.

The receptionists and clerical staff also need training, especially in the day unit's special forms of communication and information technology. The health and safety aspects of their jobs should also be taught routinely.

Summary

The scope of practice in the speciality of day surgery is continually changing and expanding. It is vital that the staff are encouraged to take advantage of the many educational opportunities available because it is only through education and research that practitioners will be equipped to offer and develop a quality service for patients. The future is likely to be less fraught if hospitals embark on planned programmes of education, research and quality assurance and day unit personnel should be trailblazers in these activities.

Key messages

(1) A day care unit is akin to a main hospital where many nurses' ambitions can be fulfilled to a gratifying extent.
(2) Supervised orientation is essential and further education needed to produce an able day care nurse.
(3) Health science colleges and day care units have much to gain by full cooperation in education programmes.
(4) Trainee nurses, operating department practitioners, receptionists and clerical staff, as well as medical and dental students all need training in day care practice.

References and further reading

Audit Commission *A Short Cut to Better Services – Day Surgery in England and Wales*, HMSO, London, 1990.

Burden, N. *Ambulatory Surgical Nursing*, W.B. Saunders, London, 1993.

National Health Service Management Executive *Day Surgery Report and Tool Kit – Report by the Day Surgery Task Force*, Health Publications Unit, Heywood, 1993.

Partridge, A.D., Brennan, M.F. and Gray, N.H. *Day Surgery – Making it Happen: A Study Conducted by the NHS Management Executive Value-for-Money Unit*, HMSO, London, 1991.

Summers, S. and Ebbert, D.W. *Ambulatory Surgical Nursing – A Nursing Diagnosis Approach*, J.B. Lippincott Company, Philadelphia, PA, 1992.

Chapter 4
Pre-assessment for Day Care

Moira Edmondson

Introduction

Pre-assessment improves the utilisation of day unit resources by screening patients for day care. It provides the opportunity, at a mutually convenient time, to assess a patient's medical and social situation before the operation. This ensures that only patients who meet the agreed criteria for admission to day surgery are chosen.

Demographic factors may affect day surgery uptake. The projected large increase of older people in the population will necessitate strict admission and discharge criteria being applied to ensure that adequate post-operative care is available following discharge from hospital. Experience has shown that if day surgery is well done there is no increased burden on community services and this is of particular concern to many family practices.

All patients admitted to the day ward for surgery under a general anaesthetic require pre-assessment, and it is also necessary for certain medical treatments, such as liver biopsy. Patients referred for procedures to be undertaken under local anaesthetic do not always require a detailed pre-assessment. A telephone interview is usually adequate, though the day surgery group for each unit will decide the protocol for this. A standard for discharge arrangements for this group of patients must be agreed and implemented.

Procedures planned for day surgery should not be such as to interfere with a patient's independence or toilet functions for a period in excess of 24 hours. Anticipated pain or nausea should be manageable with oral analgesia and antiemetics.

The nurses involved in pre-assessment clinics must be experienced and proficient in day surgery practice. They are in a key position to identify potential risks during the pre-operative interview, and can anticipate and answer any patients' or carers' questions.

Assessment is a new increased responsibility for nursing staff which should generate a joint venture with patients and facilitate medical decisions. It is deemed safe and acceptable by surgeons and anaesthetists for nurses to do this work, providing agreed strict guidelines are adhered to. The majority of patients will probably have been referred from the out-patients' clinic following a consultation with their consultant. Involvement of medical staff in pre-assessment clinics is not necessary but an anaesthetist should be readily available for advice and examination of the patient if required.

To ensure that all users are aware of the criteria used for referral of patients to the day unit an operational policy should be agreed and implemented robustly. This will require input from managers, anaesthetists, surgeons, physicians and nurses and it is recommended that each unit have a day surgery group who meet regularly (at least every three months), with representation from each professional group. These meetings agree policies and procedures and discuss any necessary changes. The group will also arbitrate with any problems between clinicians.

Pre-assessment results in well-informed patients being admitted to an environment they know about. They meet the familiar face of their named nurse and proceed through an organised day in a relaxed and comfortable manner. Relatives or friends are involved in the decision making and so are more likely to be happy with discharge arrangements and more confident about the assistance they are called on to provide at home.

It is essential that, once a patient referral is accepted, the day surgery staff manage all bookings, appointment times and admission details. Without this arrangement the risk of mistakes increases with a consequent waste of valuable resources, and the most efficient method of preventing this is to channel all bookings through the day surgery bed manager who should accept bookings under supervision of the nurse in charge. Advance bookings should be taken and time limits for these will vary according to each unit's preference, for instance bookings up to six months in advance are quite acceptable. However, pre-assessment itself should not occur more than twelve weeks before the patient's admission day, though time limits may vary from unit to unit. It is important that a minimum and maximum advance booking time be agreed and included in the operational policy, with flexibility allowed in some exceptional cases, for instance termination of pregnancy and replacement bookings may be screened the day before admission. Patients must have a minimum of two weeks' notification of their admission date so that they have enough time to organise themselves and their family. Notice of less than two weeks results in problems allocating time for pre-assessment and also leads to a higher incidence of patient cancellations, with the resulting impact on the clerical staff's time.

Patient selection

Day surgery is expanding, in terms of both the procedures which are available and the number of patients treated. It is anticipated that this growth will continue, and the day surgery nurse must ensure that the quality of care is not compromised by inappropriate referrals. Referral of patients for day surgery is ultimately a medical decision, but it is essential that a multidisciplinary approach is taken. This is especially important if the day surgery nurse has concerns based on previous experience and nursing knowledge. These should not be ignored particularly when considering that, as a result of patient satisfaction, increased demand, and negligible readmission rates, clinicians' confidence in day surgery has continually increased, with a consequence that their referrals tend to be less cautious. There is also a wide spectrum of medical and social factors that influence the referral decision.

Day surgery was initially offered only to the young and fit, but advances such as keyhole surgery and laser technology are rapidly replacing conventional methods and allow for less stressful treatment. The elderly and more complicated cases are also able to have their medical conditions controlled so that they can be safely accepted for day surgery. Modern anaesthesia facilitates uncomplicated, rapid and comfortable recovery and, as with surgical techniques, these improvements are continuous.

Notwithstanding modern advances, doctors must be assured that a decision to refer a patient for day surgery will result in a safe recovery. The risk of complication must be low, not only while the patient is in hospital but also after discharge.

Patients using the unit must first be selected using the American Society of Anesthesiologists (ASA) 1, 2 and 3 classes (see Appendix 1). Only those patients who fall into one of these classes at pre-assessment and who also satisfy local criteria, such as living within a given distance from the day surgery unit, will be treated. Providing the criteria are adhered to there is no upper age limit.

It is crucial that all patients have a choice and that they are happy to be treated as day cases if they are given the option. At preliminary selection the nature of the procedure and the routine management should be fully explained to the patient at the out-patients' consultation. (Any pathological or radiological investigations required will be undertaken at pre-assessment one or two weeks before admission.) The patient's name is added to the day surgery waiting list or the patient can be referred directly to the day surgery unit.

The majority of day wards have now designed nursing records to include nurse assessment. A nursing assessment form is a decision-making tool enabling nursing staff to arrange any investigations required or to refer patients to the medical team. Assessment clinics not only prepare patients for day surgery but must also ensure that patients who are unsuitable, either for medical or social reasons, have alternative arrangements made for their subsequent admission and treatment.

Conditions in a patient's home should enable recovery in comfort, thus an inside toilet is a necessity. There should be easy access to a telephone so that the hospital can be contacted in an emergency or for general enquiries, and the patient's journey home should preferably not take more than one hour. Experience has shown when patients are unsuitable for day surgery at pre-assessment it is most commonly due to social conditions, which other medical and nursing staff have not detected.

Booking

Advance bookings are accepted by the bed manager. The bed manager then looks at waiting lists for individual consultants and, in consultation with the day surgery manager, selects appropriate patients from lists in line with the numbers and mix of cases required for each operating theatre list.

The clerical officers send an admission letter to the patient which will include notice of the admission date and an information leaflet explaining the procedure proposed. The patient's letter will confirm the admission time and the pre-assessment date. It also gives instructions about pre-operative intake of food and drink and other general information. Patients will be advised that they need to make their own travel arrangements to and from hospital as ambulances are not available for day surgery patients, although a voluntary transport service may be available which can be arranged if requested.

All basic patient information should be sent to the day surgery clerical officers who obtain the patient notes, and collect and make ready the relevant forms and documents. Any recent blood results, X-rays and electrocardiograms must be available on the day of admission.

After acceptance of the patient for day surgery the nurse must ensure that the patient possesses and understands the written information previously sent to them. Discharge procedures should also be agreed, especially the arrangements for a responsible adult to escort the patient home and remain with them for the first 24 hours, including the first night at home. The opportunity should then be taken to introduce patients to their named nurse and to provide a visit to the ward area.

Careful consideration must be given to agreeing the admission date. It is of little use to assess patients six months before an admission date; their medical status may change as will their recall of information given. Where admission dates cannot be given less than four weeks in advance, patients should be requested to return for pre-assessment. This date should be convenient for the patient and arranged one to two weeks before their booked admission.

The assessment clinic

Correct assessment of patients for day surgery is a most important aspect for the maintenance of the quality of service within any unit. Without pre-assessment patients can experience delays and, on occasion, cancellation of their procedure. This would result in much dissatisfaction. Assessment clinics are organised by a team of nurses, and the number and grade of the team will be determined by the volume of work. The team leader may be a registered general nurse of F grade with a complement of E and D grade nurses who are experienced and deemed competent in assessment.

Assessment clinics are coordinated by the nurse in charge of the clinic in conjunction with the bed manager, who need to work closely together and establish a good communication system. If there are any contentious issues, then the day surgery manager should arbitrate. Following acceptance of bookings the bed manager is responsible for liaison with the nurse in charge to ascertain which nursing staff are available, and when. The bed manager must also inform the nurse in charge as to numbers of patients requiring evening appointments and any late bookings (due to cancellation) requiring assessment before admission. This communication is needed to provide shift patterns which are flexible and organised to ensure optimum use of the available nurses.

Assessment clinics should run on the basis that the patient is an individual who has unique circumstances. It is the first part of the 'service' and flexibility, rather than rigidity, should be a keyword. For example, many patients undergoing day surgery are young, fit and in full-time employment, and these people would probably appreciate the opportunity to attend evening clinics. The demand for such a facility can be ascertained by offering a time during normal sessions, usually 0900–1700 hrs, and then inviting patients to say if they would prefer an evening appointment, say between 1700 and 2000 hrs.

To avoid the complaint of 'conveyor belt medicine' and to foster the feeling of a caring service, at least 20 minutes should be allowed for each patient's appointment. Even an experienced nurse may require 25–30 minutes per patient. There must be time to allow patients to ask questions and air any related worries. Patients then feel that they are able to make informed decisions and have choices regarding their care. A hurried consultation will leave patients frightened and bewildered and unable to retain most of the information given to them. Continuous audit of waiting times at pre-assessment clinics must be undertaken and patients should not be waiting to be seen for more than 30 minutes after their appointment time.

When attending appointments, patients and those accompanying them should be greeted initially by the day surgery receptionist. First impressions do count greatly and a sullen, unsmiling and unhelpful receptionist in an untidy reception area is not likely to calm a nervous patient. The receptionist should show patients where they can wait and, although not essential, it is preferable to have tea and coffee available. A ready supply of magazines and books helps to pass any waiting time. The receptionist is the unit's welcoming face, but all staff should be involved and reminded of their responsibility to be aware of customer care. Here are some ways of improving service to the public.

(1) Always welcome patients with a friendly greeting and a smile.

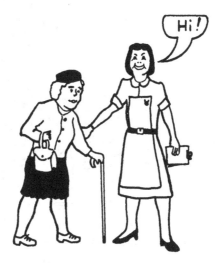

(2) Always explain to patients what they must do next and ensure they have all the information they require.

(3) Should patients require additional information, offer to obtain this. Advise patients of any anticipated delays and continue to keep them informed of what is happening.

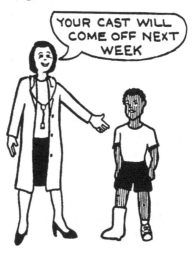

(4) Instructions must be given in a quiet environment. Speak slowly and clearly always checking patients have understood.

(5)   If things go wrong, do not ignore them: explain the problems and offer alternative arrangements wherever possible.

(6)   The area you work in should be clean and tidy. All staff should wear uniform correctly and dress smartly.

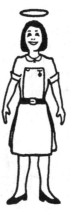

(7)   Do not leave patients to wander aimlessly. Acknowledge their presence.

(8)   If you make a mistake always recover the situation by apologising promptly.

When ready, the assessment nurse should introduce him or herself and escort the patient to the pre-assessment room. Units may like to consider allowing nurses in this role to wear mufti (tidy non-uniform), which helps the creation of a balanced relationship in which both parties have an equal footing. All patients should be seen in a private room solely for the purpose of pre-assessment. A 'do not disturb' sign should be put outside the room and at all times the patient's right to privacy should be maintained. The use of a curtain barrier is no longer acceptable, because having a history taken is very personal to each individual. All equipment required at this session should be readily available, as it shows a lack of professionalism if one constantly has to leave the room to obtain equipment. This would not instil confidence.

All nurses participating in pre-assessment should be able to perform venesection and record electrocardiograms to speed up the process and to avoid the unnecessary inconvenience of attending other departments in the hospital. Approved training should be completed prior to the nurse performing these procedures.

The nursing staff involved in pre-assessment must also have a thorough knowledge of day surgery and, in particular, the operational policy of the unit. Nursing staff must be skilled in assessment and interviewing techniques by approved training, which allows the nurse to anticipate and answer questions, but also to identify areas of potential risk. Nursing staff new to pre-assessment should not work alone for at least four weeks and should remain supervised for a further month. Audit of completed documentation must be undertaken during this period, as should patient's compliance with information given. Any cancellations on the day through failed pre-assessment must be recorded, and replacements sought by the bed manager. No cost cutting or administrative 'efficiencies' are permissable if they compromise the patient's safety.

Types of referral

The majority of day units in the UK will have one or more methods of referral. We will discuss the two most commonly used – direct referral and waiting list admissions – and review two other methods – outreach clinics and fast tracking methods. Each has its own specific advantages and disadvantages.

Direct patient referral

Direct patient referral is when patients are seen in out-patients and deemed fit for day surgery by their consultant, then sent directly to the day surgery unit for pre-assessment. These referrals are always an unknown quantity and it is usually difficult to slot them into existing pre-assessment clinics. Patients have usually been seen in a busy department, told they require surgery and asked to proceed to the day ward. After a bombardment of information they often arrive bewildered and confused (it is worth noting that patients only remember 20% of verbal information).

The distinct advantage of this method is that patients can be assessed by the nurse, receive all written information, meet their named nurse, see the day ward and be offered a date of admission convenient to them. The necessary investigations are completed and patients accept an admission date, all in one visit to the hospital.

Waiting list admission

The bed manager must hold all the relevant waiting lists. Following prior consultation and agreement with medical staff about procedures to be undertaken and numbers of patients for each list, the bed manager will select patients from the day surgery waiting list. Patients will be given an admission date and a pre-assessment appointment.

There are two inherent disadvantages to this method. First, patients are invited for pre-assessment 'blind'. Too often they are unfit for day surgery or cannot make satisfactory home arrangements. This leads to inconvenience and upset for patients and wastes valuable pre-assessment time. Clinicians should be actively encouraged to enter notes on the waiting lists of patients who are unsuitable for day case surgery, and referring surgeons should be notified in writing of the reasons for this cancellation within 48 hours. Second, a proportion of patients have often been on waiting lists for long periods of time and have decided that they no longer require treatment. There is also the group who, for whatever reason, fail to attend the pre-assessment clinic, and this leads to waste of resources.

The problem of a patient failing to attend affects many day units. To reduce this the following strategies may help:

(1) The pre-assessment nurse informs the clerical officer of any patient failing to attend for their appointment. Every effort is made to contact the patient to find the reason for non-attendance, but if clerical staff are unable to make contact a replacement is obtained.

(2) Many managers have a fear of being caught out by too many

patients attending on the same day. This is caused by overbooking or 'flying by the seat of your pants', but our experience has shown this to be a risk worth taking. There will nearly always be patients who do not attend on the appointed day of admission.

Continuous audit of failure to attend can be used as a tool to ensure that its wasteful effect is tackled.

Outreach clinics

Some consultants have recently begun to hold out-patient clinics in the evening at community surgeries. Any patient requiring day surgery is referred to the day surgery assessment nurse in attendance who will organise a pre-assessment clinic using the same guidelines that are used in the day unit. Following acceptance by the nurse, patients are then given a date of admission convenient to them, and relevant written information is handed out. However, these clinics will remain costly until more of them are established and the number of day surgery cases to be seen is known. They are not financially viable if one qualified nurse is in attendance for a full clinic session – which could last for two to three hours – and there are too few referrals (three or less).

While pre-assessment by this method is not economic, nurse-only pre-assessment clinics, held monthly and recalling patients back from previous clinics, provide an alternative. Patients at these clinics do not always meet their named nurse prior to surgery, nor do they have the opportunity to see the day ward. However, this type of referral may become more common as the emphasis on primary care grows.

Fast tracking

Fast tracking is fairly new and used in only a few centres. Patients visit their GP and are referred directly to the day unit's bed manager who places them directly onto an operating theatre list. Such patients do not see the consultant until the day on which their operation is booked, nor are they pre-assessed by a day surgery nurse. Put simply, fast-track patients form part of a back-up system in cases where other patients have been admitted to the day surgery unit and found to have unsuitable home circumstances or to be unfit for day surgery.

In the future there may be an increased demand for this method of referral as more GPs become actively involved and more experienced in its use.

It would not be unreasonable after reading the preceding paragraphs to regard pre-assessment for day surgery as problematic and difficult to organise. As with anything that is relatively new the management of change can be difficult, and it is essential that pre-assessment clinics are well managed and have a sound operational policy with clear lines of responsibility. Strict admission criteria must be adhered to in order to maintain as large a margin of safety as possible. We must accept that this policy cannot be changed at whim to accommodate a particular patient for whatever reason and it is important to remember that once a precedent is set others will expect to follow with an increased risk of complications.

Opposition to pre-assessment clinics by some clinicians still exists on the basis that this method necessitates the patient making two hospital visits, though an audit of patients in Canterbury does not show this to be a problem. On the contrary, most patients find the initial visit useful and reassuring. Many patients have fears that are based on inaccuracies and misinformation, and pre-assessment gives them the opportunity to express these fears and be reassured so as to reduce anxiety levels.

Audit of nurse pre-assessment has shown the margin of error is less than when pre-assessment is undertaken by medical staff, partly because the nurse has more time but also because medical staff may not consider the patient's social situation.

Paediatric assessment

Children should not be treated as isolated cases in an adult setting and paediatric surgery must have specific sessions or days allocated on a regular basis to meet demand. It is essential that the facilities and equipment available are of a high standard and that medical and nursing staff with paediatric experience are available. A full range of paediatric equipment must be readily available in the event of complications. Nearly all paediatric surgery requires a general anaesthetic and prior arrangements must always be made with the paediatric ward for transfer of any child requiring an overnight stay, should this be necessary.

Children will normally be in ASA classes 1 and 2 (fit with no serious disease). Children in class 3 may be suitable, but this decision must be made by a senior anaesthetist with paediatric expertise. Children under six months are not suitable for day surgery due to the possible risk of post-anaesthesia apnoea. Exceptions may be made in special hospitals for children when 'prematurity' is allowed for, that is less than 60 weeks post-conceptual.

The social circumstances of the child patient must be carefully investigated. There must be adequate facilities at home and readily available transport, and carers must be fully involved in the decisions taken as to discharge and after-care. Some parents may not wish to shoulder the responsibility of post-operative care, and their views must be respected. In these cases, alternative care should be offered.

For many children hospital admission can be very stressful and this is always minimised by involving the parents wherever possible in their care. Anxiety must also be alleviated in the parents because relaxed, informed and happy parents help produce a relaxed and happy child. A few very timid children will find a day stay, with all the associated unfamiliarity, unacceptable. They should not have their security threatened and usually benefit from a longer stay in hospital, where they should only be admitted to a paediatric ward.

Assessment of children is normally carried out in the out-patients' department. It is beneficial to staff, parents and the child if arrangements for visits to the day unit are made, and at this visit parents can be given detailed written instructions as to the fasting duration and other pre- and post-operative care. It is important they are told to inform the unit if their child develops an upper respiratory infection.

Adult pre-assessment – local anaesthesia

It is clear that patients undergoing procedures with local anaesthesia suffer the same, and often more, fear and anxiety than patients having a general anaesthetic. Yet in many units these patients are not offered the same pre-assessment. As day surgery techniques advance, more procedures are carried out without a general anaesthetic and although these patients do not require as rigorous a pre-operative assessment, patients should be given the choice of attending the unit and meeting staff. Alternatively, much can be achieved by using a telephone interview.

Telephone interview

By contacting patients by telephone a service is provided which will ensure that patients have personal contact with their named nurse. Patients are given the opportunity to ask questions and express any concerns or fears. Prior to this telephone call the patient should receive the standard admission letter and a procedure-specific information leaflet explaining that their operation is to be performed under local anaesthetic. For example, a patient who is about to have a groin hernia repaired under local anaesthetic should receive a leaflet containing the following information:

(1) Preliminary assessment arrangements, including any tests the patient may have to have.
(2) Exact attendance time, precise oral intake instructions plus medication advice. (Self shave of operation site may be requested.)
(3) Explanation of possible skin marking and local anaesthetic technique and effects.
(4) Description of early after-operation experiences. Injection or tablets for pain or nausea, wound dressing, mobilisation and refreshments. Carer requirements and travel arrangements.
(5) Home instruction, communication with family doctor, wound care, usual feelings and activities expected (including bowels, diet, discomfort, driving, sex and work).
(6) Encourage questions at any time with a direct care line.

Although it is not possible to complete a physical assessment the experienced pre-assessment nurse will be able to obtain a history over the telephone which gives clues to potential problems. Any problem patients can then be invited to attend for a pre-assessment visit. The nurse should confirm that the patient is able to provide transport to and from the unit and that, where necessary, a relative or friend is available to accompany them and look after them on their return home.

To avoid unnecessary repetition of recording and producing separate forms the documentation used for general anaesthesia should be used, using different criteria. These criteria must be agreed with the anaesthetists and members of the day surgery group.

Adult patient assessment – general anaesthetic

The patient's journey through the day surgery unit, including pre-assessment, should all be contained in one record. There are many designs used throughout the country and each unit should decide the style and format of documents necessary for their own use. This also gives the unit its own 'corporate' image. It is important that any assessment record should be reviewed annually (and changed if necessary). Ideally all users should be asked for comments so that changes can then be agreed with the day surgery group and improvements made accordingly. Surgeons and anaesthetists must jointly agree criteria for haematological investigations and agree the age above which electrocardiograms are necessary. The pre-assessment nurse will have all this information as part of the nursing standard for pre-assessment and it is the responsibility of the assessment nurse to contact medical staff for advice if any exceptions to the standards arise.

The patient's notes and any X-rays necessary should be present at the pre-assessment interview and it is the responsibility of the assessment nurse to communicate with the day surgery clerical staff to ensure that no documents are missing. It is essential that the patient's notes and all relevant documentation be available at the time of admission. There will be insufficient time on the admission day to obtain any missing paperwork. Missing documents could result in delay to the patient's surgery, or worse, the operation having to be cancelled.

Relatives and/or friends should be encouraged to be present at pre-assessment, providing the patient is happy for this to occur. It is important at this time to build a rapport with the patient, and the ambience created should be relaxed, comfortable and above all quiet. Patients should be made to feel that time is not the driving force but that the giving and receiving of information is paramount for both parties.

Operation/diagnosis

The nurse should ensure that the patient is in possession of their admission letter and procedure-specific information leaflet and should determine whether the patient's surgical problem still exists (particularly if they have been on a waiting list for some time). One may consider this unnecessary, but experience has shown patients can and do arrive on the day of admission only for medical staff to discover the original problem has resolved. This is an obvious waste of not only the patient's time but also of valuable operating theatre time.

The nurse should ensure that the patient understands exactly what procedure they are to undergo. Questions regarding this should be actively encouraged and answered simply in language the patient can understand.

Age

The age criteria used will vary. Many day units operate an upper age limit of 70. Reasons given for this are reduced mobility, covert pathology and social problems. Other units have no upper age limit providing admission/discharge criteria are met in full. Internal audit has shown that recovery time and anaesthesia-related complications are independent of age in day care patients.

A lower age limit in the day surgery unit should be set at 6 months, providing children are accommodated separately.

Past medical history

A full medical history is needed which will require the nurse to use an agreed check-list. This check-list is used for all patients requiring surgery under a general anaesthetic. The list should be agreed with the anaesthetic department where, usually, one anaesthetist is assigned to look after day surgery anaesthesia. Experience has shown that the majority of patients cancelled on the day of admission were cancelled by the anaesthetist. Their involvement in the design of and agreement to the assessment criteria is therefore crucial.

Examples of nursing documentation for pre-assessment are shown in Fig. 4.1. In the first example shown the initial five questions are clearly differentiated. The rule covering completion of this part is that any questions resulting in a 'yes' response necessitate referral to the anaesthetist on call. It then follows that the anaesthetist must decide what, if any, investigations are required, whether a consultation is required, or whether the patient's admission is cancelled/postponed. Should the latter occur, a full explanation should be given to the patient and a letter given to them to take to their GP. The assessment nurse informs the bed manager of this cancellation so that a replacement can be found whenever possible.

Patients requiring a general anaesthetic should be ASA class 1 (a normal healthy person) or class 2 (minor systemic disease which does not interfere with normal activities). Some units accept ASA class 3 (systemic disease interfering with normal activities) providing the patient's condition is controlled with or without medication. Some units use a flow chart for use by the pre-assessment nurse when deciding ASA status. A chart used by King's College Hospital, London is reproduced with permission in Fig. 4.2.

If any systemic disease is out of control, patients should be referred to the medical team. Insulin-dependent diabetics are not suitable for day case surgery under a general anaesthetic except under a set of very special circumstances.

Patients receiving oral hypoglycaemics should omit such medication on the morning of surgery. Should blood glucose levels be high or low post-operatively and/or diet and fluids not tolerated, arrangements should be made for admission overnight elsewhere and the patient and relatives informed of this.

The name of the surgeon/anaesthetist contacted and any instructions given should be noted. If appropriate these should also be recorded in the nursing notes.

Baseline observations

Temperature, pulse rate and blood pressure should routinely be recorded. Measurement of a patient's blood pressure should not be undertaken during the first five minutes of interview as a false recording may result. It is important when recording the pulse to make note of any irregularity for comparison in the event of post-anaesthetic arrthymias. Patients are usually stressed and frightened on arrival. If an abnormal recording is obtained it is advisable to take a second reading after five to ten minutes (explaining to the patient why this is necessary). If the recording remains abnormal and the diastolic blood pressure is 100 mmHg or above, medical staff should be contacted. Should this necessitate cancellation of surgery, an explanation should be given to the patient and a letter provided for their GP. The patient should be instructed to arrange a visit to their GP within seven days. If the nurse has doubts regarding the patient's compliance with these instructions it is the nurse's responsibility to contact the patient's doctor by telephone.

DAY/SHORT STAY SURGERY

Bed Number	Age
Occupation	

AFFIX

PATIENT LABEL

Pre-operative Criteria

DAY _____ DATE _____ TIME _____

CONSULTANT _____

OPERATION/DIAGNOSIS _____

DOES YOUR PROBLEM STILL EXIST?   YES/NO   If NO refer to Surgeon
Decision taken:– _____

LIST SERIOUS ILLNESSES/OPERATIONS IN THE PAST

1. _____   4. _____
2. _____   5. _____
3. _____   6. _____

PLEASE TICK CORRECT ANSWERS

		NO	YES	NURSING OBSERVATIONS
1	Do you get chest pain, palpitations on exertion?			Pulse
2	Do you get breathless or chest pain on exercise or at night?			regular/irregular
3	Do you have asthma, bronchitis or other chest disease?			
4	Do you have diabetes (sugar in the urine)?			B.P. mm hg.
5	Have you had any problems with anaesthetics? *			Wt. Kg.
6	Have you had heart disease, rheumatic fever or high blood pressure?			
7	Has any of your family had problems with anaesthetics?			Temp. C
8	Have you ever had a convulsion or fit?			
9	Have you ever had liver disease or been jaundiced?			L.M.P.
10	Do you suffer from anaemia or other blood disorders?			
11	Have you had any thrombosis?			Urine
12	Do you bleed easily or excessively?			
13	Do you get swollen ankles?			
14	Have you ever had kidney disease?			
15	Do you have a cough, cold or nose trouble?			
16	Do you have arthritis or muscle disease?			
17	Do you smoke (indicate No. per day)?			
18	Do you drink alcohol? (Indicate units per week)			
19	Do you have any known allergies (include elastoplast)?			LIST ALLERGIES HERE in RED:
20	If female, is there any possibility you could be pregnant?			_____
21	If female, when was your last menstrual period?			_____
22	Are you currently taking any drugs or other medications? (including the contraceptive pill)			_____
23	Any serious illnesses/major operations (list above)			_____
24	Caps/crowns/false teeth			

LIST DRUGS CURRENTLY TAKEN HERE:

* _____   _____

_____   _____

_____   _____

Surgeon/Anaesthetist informed?   Yes/No

Treatment:– _____   Name:– _____

_____   Signature _____

_____   Pre-assessment date:– _____

INVESTIGATIONS

BLOODS: − FBC, ECR, Gp & Save, LFTs, Glucose, ESR

Clotting _____

Other _____

Arteriogram/Angioplasty:- time _____

Localisation:- time _____

CXR _____ ECG _____

Pregnancy Test   Yes/No _____Result Pos/Neg

X-Rays requested at Pre-assessment   YES/NO

_____

_____

_____

_____

_____

_____

_____

_____

Fig. 4.1 (above and opposite) Examples of nursing documentation for pre-assessment.

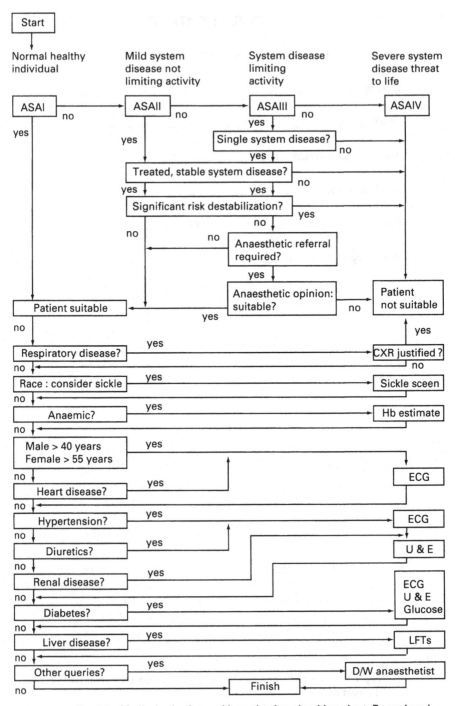

Fig. 4.2 Medical selection and investigation algorithm chart. Reproduced with permission of King's College Hospital Day Centre Staff.

All patients should have a routine urinalysis. This can be time-consuming but will help identify the undiagnosed diabetic. Any abnormalities found on routine testing are recorded and a standard letter forwarded to the patient's GP.

Obesity

A protocol for obese patients should be agreed by the day surgery group. One example is that patients should have a body mass index (BMI) of less than 34. BMI is calculated by:

$$\text{Body Mass Index} = \frac{\text{weight (kg)}}{\text{height}^2 \ (m^2)}$$

A graph of acceptable limits may be useful: that of St Bartholomew's Hospital is reproduced with permission in Fig. 4.3.

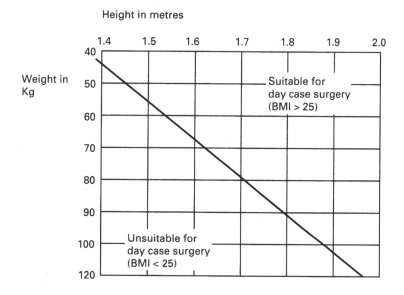

Fig. 4.3 Height–weight nomogram based on a Body Mass Index. Reproduced with permission from Van Besouw and Wilkinson.

Drugs

Patients who are receiving anticoagulant therapy should not be accepted for surgery which involves biopsy or incision. Patients taking certain drugs, diuretics for instance, may require blood chemistry to be checked. The criteria for these will have been agreed and be contained in the assessment standards. A note must be made on the front assessment sheet and the drug sheet of any drug allergies (this should be recorded in red ink). It is essential that the patient does not confuse allergies with sensitivities. For example many patients consider that nausea and gastrointestinal symptoms when taking antibiotics indicate an allergic response. Close questioning is necessary and if this proves difficult, clarification from the patient's notes or GP must be obtained.

Most patients must be told to take all their current medication as normal (unless contraindicated). Criteria for this must be agreed with the anaesthetists.

Once the medical history has been taken, the first two questions on the discharge criteria are completed. These confirm that the patient has a responsible adult to collect them and to stay with them for the first 24 hours after the operation. Unfortunately, there are patients who readily agree this arrangement only to inform the nurse at the time of discharge there is no one at home. Arrangements must be made for these patients to remain in hospital overnight (hence the value of including relatives or friends in the pre-assessment interview). Should the patient not be able to make one or both of these arrangements, the admission must be postponed and another date given if and when home circumstances are suitable. If this is not possible, the patient's admission must be cancelled and their name be added to the in-patient waiting list. (See also Chapter 7 on discharge procedure and arrangements.)

All investigations undertaken at pre-assessment should be noted on the appropriate form. It is useful to have a means available for easy attachment of all blood examination results, and the best place for these is on the reverse side of the pre-assessment questionnaire (see Fig. 4.1).

The sickle disease gene affects many ethnic groups (Afro-Caribbean, Indian and Eastern Mediterranean), so the local population factors need to be known and the sickle cell test or electrophoresis arranged accordingly. If an electrocardiogram is necessary this should be undertaken. It is the responsibility of the assessment nurse to ensure that electrocardiogram recordings are seen by medical staff prior to the patient's admission. All blood study results returned to the unit are checked against accepted normal levels. Abnormalities must be brought to the attention of the anaesthetist and, if necessary, surgery postponed or cancelled.

The assessment nurse should allow the patient a further opportunity to ask questions and ensure all written information they are given is understood. The patient and attending relatives must understand that recovery takes time and they must not expect a resumption of their normal routine at home immediately, nor indeed must it be permitted. A visit to the day surgery unit should follow with an introduction to the patient's named nurse or associate nurse wherever possible. Patients must be encouraged to telephone the day unit if they have any further queries prior to admission.

Summary

It is important to remember that patients only spend a short time in day surgery. Our objective is therefore to ensure that this time is well used to achieve the best outcome for the patient. Clear admission and discharge criteria are imperative for these objectives to be obtained.

The Royal College of Surgeons and Audit Commission have published reports on day surgery in which they recommend that patient selection be carefully considered both from the psychological and medical aspect, but also as importantly the social aspect. In both reports it is recommended that patients fulfil the criteria before their admission, therefore avoiding cancellation on the day of the operation.

To maintain the assessment nurse's credibility it is critical that all guidelines are strictly adhered to. It is futile to offer day surgery to the patient who lives alone at the top of a mountain, whose only transport is one bus a week on market day. Although this might be fanciful, patients should only be admitted and treated when they can return to an environment that enables them to fully recover safely without difficulty.

In conclusion, provided strict guidelines are formulated and adhered to, the patient's experience of day surgery will be a happy one. Many surveys show that the majority of patients find pre-assessment beneficial. It has been shown that nurses can

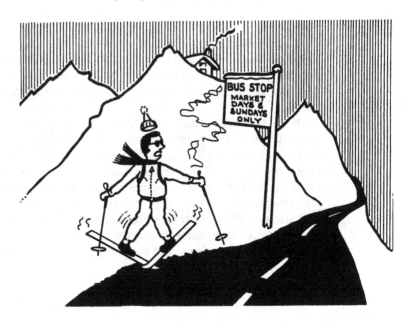

readily identify those patients who are fit and fulfil the criteria for day surgery and select those who need medical referral. This allows medical staff more time to deal with those patients who are problematic and therefore require a more in-depth assessment. Here is a final summary of the benefits of pre-assessment.

(1)   Pre-assessment allows patients to receive information and participate in the organisation of their care.
(2)   Patients meet their named nurse and familiarise themselves with the unit in the knowledge that information received has empowered them to make informed decisions in the planning of their care.
(3)   Patients feel confident knowing that help is always available by telephoning the unit.
(4)   All necessary investigations can be arranged prior to admission and results be obtained and noted.
(5)   Patients deemed unsuitable for day surgery and those who do not attend the clinic can be automatically replaced.
(6)   Patients' social circumstances are identified as suitable for day case admission and discharge.
(7)   The admission day runs smoothly resulting in patients who are less stressed and more relaxed.

Key messages

(1) Pre-assessment judges the surgical, medical, psychological and social appropriateness of patients for day care.

(2) Pre-assessment clinics allow the patient and the nurse to plan so that day care is safe and complication free.

(3) There are various referral methods which, if well structured, are equally effective.

(4) Organised pre-assessment reduces anxiety and costs through preparation and good arrangements.

References and further reading

Boyle, W. and White, P. 'Pre-operative assessment and management of adults with pre-existing problems', *Ambulatory Anaesthesia, Newsletter of the Society for Ambulatory Anaesthesia* 2, 4 (December, 1987).

Carlisle, D. 'Comic relief', *Nursing Times*, 86, 38 (1990), 50–51.

Humphreys, M.S. and Revelle, W. 'Personality, motivation and performance: a theory of the relationship between individual differences and information processing', *Psychological Review*, 91 (1984), 153–84.

Janis, I.L. and Feshbach, S. 'Effects of fear-arousing communications', *Journal of Abnormal and Social Psychology*, 48 (1953), 78–92.

Spurgeon, P. and Banwell, F. *Implementing Change in the NHS*, Chapman and Hall, London, 1991.

Swindale, J. 'The nurse's role in giving pre-operative information to reduce anxiety in patients admitted to hospital for elective minor surgery', *Journal of Advanced Nursing*, 14 (1989), 899–905.

Wilson, M., Williams, N., Baskett, P., *et al.* 'Assessment of fitness for surgical procedures and the variability of anaesthetists' judgements', *British Medical Journal*, 1 (1980), 509.

Chapter 5
Patient Information

Moira Edmondson

Introduction

The purpose of providing good information is a successful day for the patient as well as the day surgery team and it is vital that day surgery staff explain to patients what is expected of them, their relatives and their friends before, during and after their stay.

The first information about day surgery that patients receive is their diagnosis and referral, often given verbally in the distracting environment of a noisy out-patients' department and, if they are worried or in pain, it is unlikely that they will concentrate properly on what they are being told. Due to the diversity of spoken English, it is also possible that a patient may not understand verbal information because they cannot follow a nurse's or

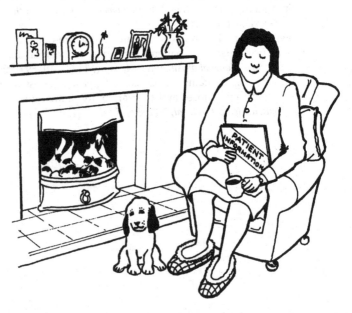

doctor's accent, and in some cases the patient may not speak English at all.

Research has shown that, in general, people only retain 20% of information given verbally, so it is unrealistic to expect patients to assimilate and understand important information about surgery, especially as the details are likely to make them feel insecure and vulnerable. Not surprisingly, most patients view their processing by the NHS to be thoroughly confusing and this is mainly due to lack of written information.

All too often, doctors and nurses consider their primary role as involvement in curative procedures and ignore the need for proper communication. In these circumstances, patients attending a day unit – either directly or from the waiting list – are likely to have forgotten verbal information, especially if it was given in a hurry. Day surgery staff should always remember that patients can be diffident about asking questions, feeling perhaps that they should not bother anyone, especially if they have been given information before.

The simplest way to ensure that patients remember information is to provide clearly written leaflets which can be referred to at any time, and especially in the safe surroundings of the patient's own home. Written patient information improves the overall level of patient satisfaction because it cuts out the anxiety

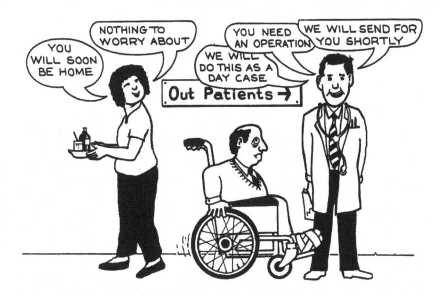

created by the unreliability of verbal information and also reduces the likelihood of increased pain which can be caused by unnecessary stress.

It has been shown that satisfied patients are more likely to follow health care instructions and this will result in greater use of health care services. More importantly, patients who are satisfied with the information and care they receive will not delay in seeking advice and will readily seek help in response to symptoms.

The information process must start at the earliest opportunity. Day surgery units with fast tracking or outreach clinics have the best control over this because the unit staff can themselves provide patients with early information, thereby ensuring that all important details are delivered in the right order and in context. The only alternative is for patients to receive written information prior to their pre-assessment interview. This comes through the patient's GP or in the out-patients' department and can result in anxiety if there is a long waiting time between referral and the pre-assessment appointment.

The content and design of this written information is crucial. As well as clear details about the unit's set-up, patients must have information that is specific to their complaint and the procedure they will undergo. Patients need to feel that they are the number one priority and day surgery units should endeavour to provide information with this point in mind. Leaflets should therefore be simple, informal (where possible) and uncrowded, because too much information crammed on to one page is confusing. A professional finish can be achieved by contracting the production of leaflets to a specialist printer.

The admission booklet

A personalised letter in the form of a booklet which gives clear instructions and is specific to the day surgery unit should be produced. This ensures that every patient receives identical information about how the unit runs and so reduces the margin for confusion. Admission letters from other departments should not be sent to patients as the day surgery unit must manage all its own admission details and use its own documents. Computer-generated mail-merge letters are also unacceptable.

The booklet should cover all details about the running of the day surgery unit, even those which might seem irrelevant, for instance experience in Canterbury showed that a significant number of patients are uncomfortable with answerphones. While there may be no alternative to having a unit answering machine, the information booklet can warn patients and perhaps give them some idea of the message they will hear. This not only prepares patients who are uncomfortable with answerphones, it results in better use of the service.

Figure 5.1 is an extract from the admission booklet developed by the day surgery unit at Kent and Canterbury Hospitals Trust and shows the kind of requests which should be made to patients at this stage. Note that reasons are given for all these requests.

(1) You must have a responsible adult to take you home and stay with you for the first 24 hours. Reflexes are slow following general anaesthetic, and you may feel tired and sleepy.

(2) You must have a shower or bath before coming to the ward. This is to ensure that the skin around the proposed operation site is clean, to reduce the risk of infection.

(3) You must remove all make-up, nail varnish and jewellery (wedding rings may be left on). The anaesthetist needs to check that oxygen levels in the blood are satisfactory. He cannot do this if you wear nail varnish and make-up.

(4) You must bring all your tablets/medicines with you, and take any medicines due on the day of operation, with sips of water (unless you have been advised otherwise). Your medicines can be taken as you do at home whilst in the ward.

(5) You must bring your nightclothes, dressing gown and toiletries. This is for your own comfort. Theatre gowns are not comfortable if worn for long periods of time.

(6) You must ring the ward if you have a cold or infection on the day before admission or, due to unforeseen circumstances, you are unable to keep your appointment. This will enable us to offer your bed to another patient and inform theatres so that theatre lists can be rearranged.

(7) Please do not bring any valuables with you, e.g. JEWELLERY, MONEY, CREDIT CARDS or CHEQUE BOOK. These may be lost or misplaced.

(8) Please do not eat any food or drink fluids after the times stated in your letter. It is not safe to administer an anaesthetic to a patient who has recently eaten or drunk.

(9) You must not drive any vehicle, drink alcohol, cook or operate machinery for 24 hours following your operation. You may feel drowsy, and reflexes are not as sharp.

(10) You must not use public transport to travel home, as this system is not always reliable.

(11) If you wish to be treated privately we can provide single rooms with en suite facilities. Please phone XXX to discuss arrangements.

Fig. 5.1 Some requests to patients in an admission booklet.

A department logo on the front cover of the booklet is a good device for helping patients identify with the day care unit, especially if the patient's name is also entered by hand on the front cover. The unit's address and telephone number should appear on the front cover, and the location should be displayed clearly in the form of a map, on the back cover, perhaps. A patient's admission date and time must be entered in a prominent place and they must receive the booklet no less than two weeks before the admission date. The booklet should also include:

- a request for patients to phone the unit to confirm their booking
- a request that patients contact the unit if the time arranged for their pre-assessment is inconvenient, in which case an alternative appointment can be made
- details about the need for either local or general anaesthesia
- a formal statement that, if patients do not follow the given instructions fully, their operation will be cancelled.

The booklet should go on to explain the quality of service patients can expect to receive and it is important that they are told who to contact if they are dissatisfied with any aspect of their care or treatment. A questionnaire to assess patient satisfaction should be included along with an explanation of how to fill it in, and a regular audit of completed questionnaires should be undertaken. Patients whose questionnaires express dissatisfaction with the service they received should be invited back to the unit to discuss their problems (see Chapter 9 on follow-up arrangements).

To complete the admission booklet, there must be some general information for patients and carers. This will be tailored for each unit, but Fig. 5.2 shows the kind of information which day surgery patients in Canterbury found useful.

The information folder

An information folder is an attractive addition to any day unit and is not unlike the glossy brochures in hotel rooms which tell guests about the hotel's facilities. Day surgery units are strongly advised to produce such a folder which they can place on every bedside locker and in the unit's waiting areas.

General Information

Information folders are situated on each bedside locker and in the waiting area. These give details of the facilities available in the day surgery suite and within the hospital.

(1) Relatives and friends are welcome to stay with you and visit at any time.
(2) Drink machines are provided in waiting areas. These facilities are free for patients. Relatives and friends may use this at a cost of 30p per drink.
(3) Restaurant and shop facilities are available on the ground floor.
(4) Ambulances are not available for use. However, the voluntary car service is. Please ask your nurse for more information. There is a charge for this service.
(5) Beds and trolleys are accommodated in single sex bays.
(6) Please phone XXX to confirm your booking. Your relatives may use XXX to contact the ward for general enquiries.
(7) You may not have your operation or procedure immediately after your admission time. You may wish to bring books/magazines with you to read while you are waiting.
(8) Patients having their operation/procedure under local anaesthetic will remain awake during this. It is advisable to have someone to accompany you home. Your nurse will advise you.
(9) The hospital operates a No Smoking policy, which I am sure you will understand is for the benefit of all.

Fig. 5.2 General information for patients before day care.

The folder includes specific inserts which can be removed and replaced where required. Figure 5.3 shows a possible list of contents for an information folder, and examples of actual inserts are given in Appendix II.

Figure 5.3 has a copy of the consent form as the last item on the list. Things happen quickly on admission day and patients should be directed to look at this copy as soon as possible, otherwise they may not see the form until the doctor arrives, explains the operation and requests the patient's signature on the consent form; a consent which can hardly be informed under such speedy circumstances.

Procedure-specific information leaflets

The list of 20 common day surgery procedures listed by the Audit Commission in 1990 has been superseded and there are now

```
┌─────────────────────────────────────────────────────────┐
│                         INDEX                            │
│                                                          │
│  • Welcome to your ward        • Private medical forms/  │
│  • The ward team                 refund of expenses      │
│  • Your named nurse            • Your consent form       │
│  • Your bed area               • Pre-operative care/your │
│  • Ward seating area             operation               │
│  • Daily ward routine          • Post-operative care     │
│  • Visiting                    • Discharge advice        │
│  • Car parking                 • Hospital chaplaincy services │
│  • Smoking                     • The Patient's Charter rights │
│  • Meals                       • Access to medical/nursing │
│  • Tea, coffee and beverages     records                 │
│  • Toilets and bathrooms       • Alternative medicine    │
│  • Public telephone            • Fire procedure          │
│  • Hospital shops              • Quality assurance       │
│  • Pharmacy services           • Breast care service     │
│  • Financial services          • Copy of consent form    │
└─────────────────────────────────────────────────────────┘
```

Fig. 5.3 Example of an index from a patient information folder.

many other medical procedures and operations commonly carried out in day care. As the list expands, day care units must invest adequate time and money producing information leaflets specific to all the procedures they carry out.

In any medical environment different patients are often given different instructions, and post-operative advice sometimes depends entirely on which doctor is performing the surgery. This can be a major obstacle to producing good information leaflets, but with the influence of the day surgery working group, the basic content of the leaflets can be agreed. (The day surgery working group is made up of representatives from the local community who have an understanding of the community and of day surgery issues. They perform a similar function to a parent governor in a school.) The leaflets produced should then be used by patients for no more than six months, during which time a continuous audit of patients', clinicians', nurses' and managers' views should be taken and necessary amendments made to the leaflet for the following six months. Every user of the unit must be involved or the agreement on suitable advice has little hope for survival.

Copies of all the available information leaflets should be displayed on the walls in the unit, and all new medical and nursing staff must become conversant with their content.

It might be tempting to group various procedures together or to produce separate information leaflets for general and local anaesthetic, but it is more important to provide clear, specific information. However minor the procedure might seem to the staff, for the patient it is major and also very personal. If a patient has been told that they are to have a sigmoidoscopy, it would be very confusing to receive a leaflet entitled:

'Sigmoidoscopy/EUA/Manual dilation of Anus GA/LA'

On seeing this leaflet the patient might think they are to have three or maybe even four procedures, or that they did not understand what they were told in out-patients. So, while the individual procedure leaflets have common sections, each one must be unique and the front cover should have a clear, simple statement telling the patient that the leaflet is for their procedure.

The information that patients receive must be produced in a style that is pleasing to the eye, easy to understand and easy to read. The relevant leaflet(s) should be sent out with the admission booklet or, if the patient has been referred directly to the day unit, given to them by hand, also along with the admission booklet.

Examples of two procedure-specific leaflets – one surgical and one medical – are given in Appendix III. It is worth noting that the heading 'Welcome to your ward' is in bold while the description of the procedure is kept to a shortish paragraph so as not to invite confusion or fear. Clear information about diet and drugs is provided, along with details about how the day unit will orchestrate the procedure. Instructions which patients have already read in the admission booklet are reiterated, for instance 'DO NOT use public transport'.

Each day care unit will have to adapt these leaflets to reflect their own practice, but the two examples provide guidelines for the sort of information which must be included. Units should also consider providing drug leaflets which are specific for the medication that patients have been given to take home (these will most commonly be analgesics). The leaflet must include a help-line number with the name of the person who usually answers the phone. Advice on producing drug information leaflets should be sought from the pharmacy department, but the style and content should be in keeping with other information leaflets. An example of a drug leaflet is reproduced in Appendix IV.

For procedures such as termination of pregnancy or breast surgery, patients may require special counselling. An extra information sheet may be required for this and an example is the Breast Care Service leaflet, given in Appendix II.

Ensuring access to the information

There are always patients who do not or will not read information given to them. This is a singularly difficult problem to solve, but a brief summary of contents often helps, in which the most important information is given in bullet points and the reluctant patient's attention drawn to these by day surgery staff. It is also a good idea to encourage relatives and friends to read and understand the content of leaflets, as they can then pass on any information which the patient might have missed. There are alternatives to written information leaflets, such as audio tapes and videos, but units can only afford to produce a handful so they have to be more general and cannot give specific information quickly. The patient consequently has to spend time locating the relevant section. Furthermore, the tapes may not be available at discharge when the patient needs more information and loaning the tapes out could prove costly if they are not returned.

A list of people who are skilled and willing interpreters of the prevalent local languages should be kept in the day care unit so that they can be called upon as needed, and these individuals may need training in the terminology relevant to specific procedures. Staff in the day unit should have a basic knowledge of communicating with deaf people so that they can pass on any essential verbal instructions, and audio tapes of the information leaflets should be made for use by blind people. Day surgery staff should also know who to contact for expert advice when dealing with patients with learning difficulties. Above all, patients with special needs of any kind need extra care to ensure that they understand the necessary information.

Admission day

On admission day, all the information about a patient must be available to staff, while patients need to have information verified for them and about them.

The clerical staff have a vital role to play in ensuring a smooth and efficient service for patients on admission day and to ensure this the unit's receptionist and nursing staff must have a list of all patients expected on that day. Staggered admission times are advisable as they give the receptionist an opportunity to have more personal contact with patients when they arrive, for instance to greet them by name. Clerical staff should produce up-to-date theatre lists for nursing staff and must inform nurses of any late cancellations or non-attending patients so that lists can be amended and theatres informed. Patients' notes, X-rays and relevant blood tests must also be made available by the clerical staff.

The named nurse verifies the patient's identity verbally and then formal identification is provided by means of an identification bracelet on which any drug allergies should be clearly displayed. The use of multiple ID bracelets for this purpose will depend on the policy of the individual unit.

During the admission interview, patients will be asked if there have been any changes in their medical status since pre-assessment and it is particularly important to establish whether a patient has developed an upper respiratory infection. If they have such an infection, their procedure will be cancelled. The nurse must also confirm arrangements for discharge and after-care with the patient and accompanying relatives or friends. If, for whatever reason, the patient cannot meet the discharge criteria, arrangements must be made for acceptable overnight accommodation, and if these cannot be made the procedure must be cancelled.

If the patient is taking regular medication, the nurse must check that it has been taken (unless the patient was instructed otherwise).

Patients will have been given instructions about the intake of food and drink, and the nurse needs to check that these have been followed. It is not enough to ask a patient when they last had something 'by mouth' as the majority of patients assume this refers only to food. If the nurse is in any doubt about the patient's compliance with instructions, the anaesthetist must be informed. Those patients admitted to the unit who have not followed advice about bathing should be requested to do so after hair has been removed from the operation site. It is also important that the nurse takes note of any abrasions of the skin and any existing pressure sores.

All information gathered must be noted in a way that is easy to read. Each part of the patient's journey through the unit is to be recorded by an individual nurse so that there is clear evidence of the responsible parties in the event of any problems. Careful noting also facilitates audit.

Patient dignity

The patient's privacy and dignity are to be guarded at all times and a supply of constant reassuring information is the first step to ensuring this.

When patients are interviewed on admission, a private room must be available for confidentiality to be maintained. Patients will sign the consent form for their procedure during this interview and may require physical and emotional support around this time, so wherever possible the named nurse should remain with the patient at this time. Relatives and friends must not be excluded at admission because they provide excellent support, and if they are not at the medical interview they should be reunited with the patient soon afterwards. They can be directed to the unit's waiting area when they cannot actually be with the patient and should be told how to find the hospital cafeteria for meals. Tea, coffee, and maybe snacks too, should be available in the unit itself.

Where clinicians insist on all undergarments being removed, the use of disposable underwear is desirable to help patients keep their dignity intact. Patients must be told where and when to change their clothes, and how to wear an operating theatre gown. A personal locker, cupboard or container should be provided for clothes and personal belongings which, ideally, will be a mobile unit that is taken to the patient's recovery area and will have been secured with a key. Patients should be encouraged to leave valuables with relatives or friends but, if they must be stored by the unit, the hospital's safety policy must be adhered to.

There is some controversy about the need for patients to remove make-up and nail varnish. Staff should be aware of individual clinicians' views on the issue and act accordingly. Any patients who need to remove make-up should be asked to do so on admission, as it is humiliating to be told of this regulation only on arrival in the operating theatre.

Wherever possible, patients who wear glasses, a hearing aid or dentures should be allowed to keep wearing them until anaesthetic induction. This will make them feel more confident and it also ensures good communication. These aids are returned to the patient as soon as possible.

Many patients have a fear of needles. Where this is apparent, the nurse can warn the medical staff who may prescribe a local anaesthetic cream which must be applied in enough time to take effect before the procedure, and if a pre-medication has been prescribed it must be given at the right time as it is of little benefit if the patient receives sedation only five minutes before surgery. Patients who are particularly nervous about their operation should be scheduled to go into the operating theatre as early as possible after their arrival. Any drugs prescribed by medical staff must be given as scheduled and, before administration, the nurse must ensure that the patient has no sensitivity or allergy to the drug they are about to receive.

Summary

The admitting nurse in day surgery is responsible for ensuring there have been no oversights at pre-assessment and that the patient's notes and all necessary information are available on the day.

Any patient coming to the day unit who has not undergone pre-assessment must first have this done and such patients should be admitted early on the morning or afternoon of their planned operation to allow time.

The smooth flow of patients safely and efficiently through the day unit hinges on a factual and reliable pre-assessment which has built-in systems for cross-checking. Without this the day will be chaotic and stressful for both patient and staff.

Key messages

(1) Good information empowers patients to prepare fully for day care.
(2) Agreement on the wording of pamphlets should be confirmed by all concerned so that they are authoritative.
(3) Procedure-specific advice is preferred because broad statements confuse.
(4) Professional design and printing improve customer appeal.

References and further reading

Crotty, M. 'Communication between nurses and their patients', *Nurse Education Today*, 5 (1985), 130–34.

Dunbar, J.M. and Agras, W.S. 'Compliance with medical instructions', in: Ferguson, J.M. and Taylor, C.B. (eds) *The Comprehensive Handbook of Behavioural Medicine*, vol. 3, Lancaster MTP Press, 1980, 115–45.

Engstrom, B. 'The patient's need for information during hospital stay', *International Journal of Nursing Studies*, 21 (1984), 113–30.

French, K. 'Methodological considerations in hospital patient opinion surveys', *International Journal of Nursing Studies*, 18 (1981), 7–32.

Ley, P. 'The psychology of compliance', in: Chourne, D.J., Gruneberg, M.M. and Eiser, J.R. (eds) *Research in Psychology and Medicine*, vol. 2, Academic Press, London, 1979, 187–202.

Mills, J. and Aronson, E. 'Opinion change as a function of the communicator's attractiveness and desire to influence', *Journal of Personality and Social Psychology*, 1 (1965), 173–7.

Moores, B. and Thompson, A.G.H. 'What 1357 hospital patients think about aspects of their stay in British acute hospitals', *Journal of Advanced Nursing*, 11 (1986), 86–102.

National Health Service Management Executive, Value for Money Unit *Day Surgery – Making it Happen*, HMSO, London, 1991.

Riley, C.S. 'Patient's understanding of doctor's instructions', *Medical Care*, 4 (1966), 34–7.

Chapter 6
Day Surgery Perioperative Concerns
Sarah Penn

Introduction

The principles of patient care in a day surgery operating theatre are essentially the same as those for patients who are cared for in any operating theatre. The theatre nurse may act as the patient's advocate during a period when the patient has little or no control, depending on the type of anaesthesia, and the nurse must therefore be aware of the patient's safety, privacy and dignity. For the day surgery nurse to become competent in operating theatre nursing techniques, specific education and training courses should be undertaken as described in Chapter 3.

This chapter highlights the differences between practice in day surgery and in-patient operating theatres. Furthermore patient care in the endoscopy room will also be discussed and many of the issues addressed may be relevant to areas such as out-patient clinics, GP surgeries performing minor surgery, laser treatments and endoscopies.

Perhaps the key features of a day surgery unit are a rapid, high volume throughput, a variety of anaesthetic techniques, involving local and regional anaesthesia under sedation, and the need for the astute day surgery theatre nurse to ensure that patients are discharged shortly after surgery and anaesthesia, according to strict discharge criteria. In-patient nurses do not have these total responsibilities and it is most important that day units are appropriately staffed by trained nursing staff and not by occasional in-patient theatre nurse visitors.

Psychological factors

The day surgery patient will arrive in the procedure room or operating theatre having been prescribed no pre-medication.

Many good day units produce excellent perioperative patient information and patients value these referral documents. Since many day cases will be apprehensive and anxious prior to surgery and anaesthesia, the efficient day surgery nurse will have to allocate time for allaying these fears (see Chapter 5). Despite this, many patients remain fearful and this is where excellent patient communication should be fostered by the theatre nurses or the operating department practitioners (ODPs).

As in the USA many British day units do not have a separate anaesthetic room. This is considered acceptable practice and is not a problem if patients are told beforehand that they will walk straight into the theatre accompanied by an ODP or nurse. However, it is essential that both medical and nursing staff vacate the operating theatre before the patient enters, leaving just the anaesthetist to welcome the patient. It is important to maintain a calm theatre environment with minimal equipment and sterile instrument trolleys around. Certainly, in teaching hospitals there is no place for a group of medical students and postgraduates to receive their teaching while an anxious patient enters the theatre.

Patients should continually be kept informed of what is being done to them until general anaesthesia is induced, and nurses may be required to communicate with day patients should the operative procedure be performed under local or regional anaesthesia. For instance the application of a blood-pressure cuff or diathermy plate may be disconcerting for a patient, especially if they are expecting another area of the body to be prepared for surgery. Applying cold cleaning fluids unexpectedly to any operative site may make the patient move involuntarily, thereby enhancing anxiety. A familiar nurse or ODP who has already established patient rapport should stay with the patient to instil confidence throughout either the induction of general anaesthesia or the performance of local or regional anaesthetic techniques. Nurse continuity is a most important aspect of day surgery practice.

An awareness by all personnel in the operating theatre of noise levels and professionalism should be maintained. This will be essential for patients undergoing local or regional anaesthesia or sedation, but is equally important during general anaesthetic induction. General anaesthesia is often maintained at adequate levels to assist post-operative recovery, and it is important to remember that hearing is the last sense to be altered and the first to recover in the recovery area. All staff handling unconscious patients under anaesthesia or sedation should be aware that patients may hear nursing comments in the operating theatre and, with an increase in litigation in the UK, great care should be taken to avoid flippant remarks.

Again the 'scrub' nurse should bear these conversational issues in mind, especially if the patient is conscious during surgery. The 'scrub' nurse should be proficient and able to anticipate the surgeon's needs without having to wait to be asked for instruments because patient anxiety levels will increase if the surgeon has to demand a knife, especially since many patients will be covered with drapes and will therefore be unable to see what is happening. Good rapport and sign language should be developed between the 'scrub' nurse and her surgical colleagues.

Transporting patients to the operating theatre

Prior to surgery, many day cases will be gowned up and taken to a waiting area. This area should be away from the busy admission room and care should be taken with patient facilities to ensure decor, music and reading are appropriate.

A nurse or ODP should collect the patient from the pre-operative area. When collecting any patient, staff should remove face masks so that they reduce any barriers to communication. The nurse or ODP then has the responsibility to check the patient's name, hospital identity number, medical record, consent form and proposed operation. Great care should be taken to identify the patient's operative site. It cannot be overstressed that, even in the best of day units, errors may happen. The nurse or ODP collecting pre-operative day cases must adopt a safety check routine. They should bear in mind that patients are frequently stressed and may reply with great conviction to a false name. Patient identity bands should be read and checked against the notes.

There are various methods used to transport patients to the operating theatre. In some day units patients walk unaided into the theatre and climb on to a conventional operating table. In others, operating trolleys are used to eliminate the need to transfer patients after surgery, while in those day units where the pre-operative area is some distance from the operating theatre, conventional trolleys are used for patient transport. Whichever mode is used the escort will need to maintain the patient's comfort and dignity during the transfer and positioning on the operating table. There is no excuse for allowing operating theatre gowns to open at the back. Such an action only serves to produce heightened patient anxiety and subsequent loss of self-esteem.

Analgesia

Nursing staff will appreciate that several day case operations are indeed painful, for instance hernia repair, varicose vein surgery, laparoscopic sterilisation, circumcision and bilateral bat ear correction. At Addenbrooke's Hospital, an analysis of 40,000 day cases revealed an overall in-patient admission rate of 1%, that is just 400 cases. Pain and post-operative nausea and vomiting were the main factors. Pre-emptive analgesia (pain relief prior to painful stimulation) has its proponents but current clinical evidence of its efficacy is lacking.

On the induction of general anaesthesia many anaesthetists administer intravenous fentanyl, alfentanil or sufentanil. These synthetic opiates produce few post-operative side-effects and this analgesia should be backed up with local anaesthetic blocks. For instance 10 ml bupivacaine 0.75% plain is ideal for reducing post-laparoscopic pain, and the use of long-acting local anaesthetic (0.25–0.75%) for, say, hernia blocks is strongly recommended.

Non-steroidal anti-inflammatory drugs (NSAIDs) such as diclofenac, ketorolac and ibuprofen are also commonly used in day surgery. These drugs may reduce the requirements for opiates in day surgery, thereby producing minimal post-operative sequelae.

All staff working within a day surgery environment should be aware that certain operations do produce significant pain and that drugs are freely available to alleviate such pain. Audit of analgesia within a day unit is an important contribution to patient care and the nursing staff should be prime movers in pain relief, for instance the 'scrub' nurse should always have bupivacaine on her trolley. There is a need for new drug delivery systems, especially in the home environment, and progress has been made with transdermal patches, sublingual analgesia and continuous subcutaneous infusion systems. All day unit staff should endeavour to treat pain effectively whether the day patient is in the operating theatre, recovery or main ward area. There is no excuse for poor pain relief and nursing staff should remember the effectiveness of paracetamol, soluble aspirin, codeine and NSAID suppositories.

Anaesthesia

Many surgical procedures are the same whether they are performed on in-patients or day cases. However, anaesthetic techniques may differ and advances in new anaesthetic agents have had a major impact on the expansion of day surgery practice. One of the essential features of good day case anaesthesia is a swift return to street fitness. Nowadays intravenous and general inhalational anaesthetics are of the highest standard, thereby making this goal attainable.

In Britain the most commonly used intravenous anaesthetic induction agent in day units is undoubtedly propofol. At Addenbrooke's Hospital a recent audit indicated that 98% of all day case anaesthetics involved the administration of intravenous propofol for induction. Critics of the drug stress that it is expensive, but the rapid, clear-headed recovery with propofol produces quality anaesthesia. There is minimal post-operative nausea and vomiting (PONV), allowing patients to be discharged after a short recovery period. Indeed, the hotel costs of admitting patients to hospital are minimised and this is inevitably the result of propofol use. The lack of PONV with this drug will decrease overall costs because antiemetics are not required and nursing time is saved.

General anaesthesia is maintained either by inhalational agents or by total intravenous anaesthesia (TIVA). The latter is a technique using propofol with an analgesic agent such as alfentanil which, after the bolus injection to induce anaesthesia, is continued either by intermittent injection or with the use of a syringe pump. For personnel in the operating theatre and recovery area, TIVA has a great advantage over the inhalational agents because it produces no pollution hazards, though two inhalational anaesthetics – sevoflurane and desflurane – have recently been introduced into British day care practice. Gaseous induction with sevoflurane makes it useful for children, while desflurane provides quicker recovery times – alas with more PONV.

The Brain laryngeal mask airway has altered anaesthetic practice and this device, used with propofol, has an established place in day surgery anaesthesia. Reports have been published about the use of the laryngeal mask airway in laparoscopic gynaecological surgery with spontaneous breathing. This technique avoids the risks of endotracheal intubation and muscle pains from the use of relaxants.

Children and adults with a needle phobia may find the use of a eutectic mixture of local anaesthetic (EMLA) cream 30–60 minutes before induction of anaesthesia produces painless venous cannulation. To maximise the benefit of EMLA, it may be necessary on paediatric lists to apply the cream to the first patient's hand before the arrival of the anaesthetist. If this is the case, a formal prescribing policy for the application of EMLA should be drawn up with the agreement of the anaesthetists. This is just another example of how the nursing staff in a busy day unit may work effectively within a multidisciplinary team.

Post-operative nausea and vomiting (PONV)

Post-operative nausea and vomiting has a detrimental effect on the success of any day unit as it can prove expensive and may lead to an increased hospital admission rate. Chapter 8 discusses this issue in detail, but the precautions listed below may reduce the incidence of PONV. Anaesthetists need to identify and pro-phylactically treat those patients at high risk.

(1) At pre-operative screening patients with a previous history of motion sickness and/or PONV following previous sur-gery should have these factors highlighted on their care plans so that the anaesthetist may prescribe and administer antiemetics.

(2) Care should be taken when moving patients, both during anaesthesia and in the recovery period. There is no merit in a hasty post-operative recovery period, and day cases should be allowed to recover naturally. Patients should therefore not be moved quickly and they benefit from being sat up gradually.

(3) Pharyngeal suction in the operating theatre and the recovery area should be kept to a minimum.

Day case nursing staff should remember that PONV may be decreased if prompt antiemetic therapy, such as ondansetron, metaclopramide, droperidol or ephedrine is considered. Again, nurses play a major role in the continual auditing of PONV and experience has shown that it is a multifactorial problem.

The role of the 'scrub' nurse

The 'scrub' nurse's role is the same as in any operating theatre, but throughout surgery nurses should remember that the patient will soon be discharged to their own home. As previously mentioned, excellent communications should occur with other team members, especially if patients have undergone local or regional anaesthesia, and concise instructions should also be given with regard to the treatment of post-operative pain and PONV.

With the rapid patient turnover, extra care should be taken by the 'scrub' nurse or ODP to ensure that the right patient has been brought to theatre for the correct operation on the appropriate site. Time should be taken to check the consent form, the patient's identity band and any allergies to prevent mishaps. Nurses should be aware that there is a higher risk of medical errors in a busy day surgery unit, but that good training and teamwork should prevent disasters.

The 'scrub' nurse should also consider the provision of correct wound care. In day surgery wound drains should be avoided unless absolutely necessary, but if required the type of drain and the length of time it is needed should be planned. A small vacuum drain may be used and can often be removed before the patient is discharged from the day unit. Wound dressings should be selected carefully, remembering that where possible the patient should be able to care for them without having to rely on community nursing staff, and the 'scrub' nurse should attempt to make dressings as simple as possible. For example, if a patient needs a pressure dressing following their procedure, a wound dressing should be applied directly on to the wound, with the pressure dressing over it. This enables the patient to remove the pressure the following day without disturbing the wound itself.

Immediate post-operative recovery

Recovery is divided into three phases and the day unit nurse will be involved with the immediate and delayed recovery period prior to patient discharge. Recovery nurses should have the same skills as an in-patient recovery nurse, and they ought to be conversant with the effects of different anaesthetic techniques, pain relief and PONV issues. Careful monitoring of the patient needs to be maintained until the patient has regained consciousness, and the parameters routinely measured are the skin colour, pulse, blood pressure and arterial oxygen saturation.

Children must be protected from injury with padded trolley rail covers and should be reunited with their parents or carers as soon as possible after they awake.

Health and safety

National and local guidelines on all issues related to health and safety must be adhered to and regular audits should be maintained to ensure safe practice. Every member of the team has a responsibility to participate in identifying areas of risk and ensuring that they are evaluated and controlled. Each unit ought to consider the surgical procedures undertaken, the equipment and substances used, policies and practices, and the educational needs of staff to minimise risk, for instance some units use lasers for particular procedures and these require particular safety precautions. Methods of reducing risk must be continually updated as new practices and procedures evolve, new equipment is purchased, patient documentation is altered and new members of staff join the team. A regular (at least monthly) check on identified areas of risk ought to be undertaken to ensure safe practice. Are entries in patient documentation legible, signed and dated? Are hazards such as sharps boxes out of the reach of children? Is the unit clean? Are two people manoeuvering patient trolleys? Especially in the operating theatre, but in other areas as well, regular maintenance of equipment should be carried out.

This book cannot address the health and safety of a day surgery unit in proper detail, as it merits an entire volume to discuss it in depth. The aim is to highlight the importance of risk management, to encourage the reader to seek professional help from their own Trust's risk management officer and to study the subject much more thoroughly.

Endoscopy

Many day surgery units also incorporate a vast range of endoscopic investigations and therapies. As with operating theatre practice this book does not attempt to address endoscopy nursing and endoscopic techniques in any detail. However, it is hoped that by reading this book endoscopy nurses will benefit from applying the same nursing principles such as:

- patient information and education
- care of the patient in the procedure room
- the need to monitor patients' vital signs
- patient recovery and discharge

- management issues, such as booking procedures
- quality issues.

Conclusion

The responsibilities of the theatre, recovery- or procedure-room nurse during the patient's perioperative period are becoming increasingly demanding. The criteria for suitable patients and the procedures that are carried out in the day surgery setting are being extended. Education and the need to maintain skills will be paramount to the success of all day units.

Day patients who are hospitalised for short periods have a right to expect expert care. Day surgery units must employ a high proportion of experienced nurses who are capable of working across all areas of the unit. If quality medical and nursing care is to be provided for day cases, Trusts will have to allocate adequate resources for patient care, audit, education and research. Throughout Britain there is evidence that health authorities have been slow to adopt these policies, and yet by the year 2000 it has been projected that day surgery will account for 60% of all elective surgery. A serious review of all future nursing policies is therefore respectfully invited.

Key messages

(1) For the physiological and psychological care of patients perioperatively the adage 'do unto others as one would have done' is most apt.

(2) While pain, nausea and vomiting are primarily post-operative matters their origin often depends on previous attention.

(3) The operating- and endoscopy-room nurse is a technician for set procedures who is closely involved with total day care of patients.

References and further reading

Bradshaw, E.G. and Davenport, H.T. *Day Care – Surgery, Anaesthesia and Management*, Edward Arnold, London, 1989.

Burden, N. *Ambulatory Surgical Nursing*, W.B. Saunders, London, 1993.

Healy, T.E.J. *Anaesthesia for Day Case Surgery*, Baillière Tindall, London, 1990.

Ogg, T.W. and Watson, B.J. *Anaesthesia Rounds – Aspects of Day Surgery and Anaesthesia: A Multidisciplinary Approach*, Zeneca Pharmaceuticals, Medicine Group Education Ltd, Abingdon, 1995.

The Royal College of Surgeons of England *Guidelines for Day Case Surgery* (revised edition), Royal College of Surgeons, London, 1992.

Summers, S. and Ebbert, D.W. *Ambulatory Surgical Nursing – A Nursing Diagnosis Approach*, J.B. Lippincott Company, Philadelphia, PA, 1992.

Thornes, R. *Just for the Day: Children Admitted to Hospital for Day Treatment*, NAWCH Ltd, London, 1991.

Wetchler, B.V. *Anesthesia for Ambulatory Surgery*, 2nd edn, J.B. Lippincott Company, Philadelphia, PA, 1991.

Whitwam, J.G. *Day-Case Anaesthesia and Sedation*, Blackwell Scientific Ltd, Oxford, 1994.

Chapter 7
Discharge Procedure and Arrangements

Moira Edmondson

Introduction

The planning and preparation for discharge of day surgery patients should begin immediately after selection and referral to the day unit. Patients can find out the arrangements they need to make for discharge at the pre-assessment clinics and from written information they are given. The pre-assessment nurse and the patient share responsibility in deciding if the patient's home circumstances will allow the patient to recover safely in the comfort of their own home. In addition, it is the nurse's professional responsibility to ensure continuity of care after the patient is discharged, using external agencies, such as district nurses, if necessary.

Discharge criteria and nursing standards must be formally agreed by the day surgery working group and strictly followed. The criteria, which will vary in individual units, should be regularly audited and if an audit shows persistent problems the criteria must be reviewed. At all times consideration must be given to any legal implications. The criteria should be concise, comprehensive and applicable to all patients and procedures carried out within the unit. Written discharge information for the patient and a carers' information leaflet for relatives or friends will contribute to a consistency of care.

Deciding when a patient is fit for discharge is fundamentally the responsibility of the clinicians and, again, the criteria they use to make this decision vary across the country. Some units insist that every patient must be seen by a doctor before leaving, while in others, doctors discharge the patient following the early recovery phase. In many units the final decision is taken by nursing staff who either follow predetermined criteria or confer with medical staff by telephone about the patient's fitness for discharge. However, nurse discharge can only be practised where units have a strong multidisciplinary approach and there is mutual regard between medical staff and nurses. If the nurse is in any doubt as to the patient's fitness for discharge, or the patient does not fulfil the discharge criteria, medical staff must be contacted directly, their advice sought and appropriate action taken and documented. Nurse discharge from the day unit speeds the process for patients, as medical staff are all too often busy elsewhere and not immediately available.

Safe discharge of day surgery patients for continuing care must be carried out by experienced and well-trained staff. Nurses must only undertake this role when they have received relevant training and have the confidence to act independently without supervision.

It is difficult to describe a typical post-operative recovery. Each patient reacts differently because there are many things which affect the process of recovery. Some of these are listed below.

- the general health of the patient
- the age of the patient
- the patient's pain threshold, pre-medications given and other drugs regularly taken
- the quality of written information given prior to surgery
- drugs used by the anaesthetist
- the patient's reaction to anaesthetic
- the activity of the unit and staffing levels
- the expertise of the anaesthetist
- the standard of pre-assessment
- the patient's perception of expected recovery time
- the occurrence of any perioperative accident.

All or some of these factors may affect the patient's arousal and recovery time. This list, though not exhaustive, indicates that patients can only be discharged when their individual physical and psychological condition allows and that their discharge cannot be to any predetermined timetable. Patients and relatives must understand the probable differences in recovery time between patients because problems arise when patients feel they are not recovering as well as expected. The following description of an occurrence in our day unit in the Kent and Canterbury Hospital helps illustrate this point.

Three men were admitted to the day unit for repair of their inguinal hernias under local anaesthetic. All three had received identical written information and were pre-assessed by a nurse. Following surgery all appeared to make a straightforward recovery and were discharged home, but during an audit of questionnaires we noticed that one of these patients had noted that he was unhappy to go home and felt he was discharged too soon. This patient was invited to attend a quality review meeting where, to our astonishment, he revealed that it was himself rather than the nursing staff who had precipitated his discharge. As stated, he was admitted with two other patients for the same type of operation, both of whom recovered quickly, got up and were ready to go home. Our third patient understandably felt that he too should be at the same stage of recovery and so, despite being in pain, feeling weak and sick, he convinced nursing staff that he was well and keen to go home. He was therefore discharged home where he spent a very uncomfortable night. Interestingly when telephoned the day after his operation, this patient still did not complain that he had any problems.

One could argue that an observant and experienced day surgery nurse should have realised that this patient was having difficulties or that stringent discharge criteria should have prevented him from leaving the unit. However, it is important to accept that it can be very difficult to identify such problems if patients are unwilling to divulge the truth.

Each unit will have a minimum recovery time for patients following surgery under general anaesthetic, for example three hours. This time may need to be extended if opiates are given and protocols must be agreed with the anaesthetists.

Additional discharge criteria are required for certain procedures and these will be agreed with individual clinicians. For example, after epidural anaesthesia patients must regain full use of lower limbs and have voided urine, and following termination of pregnancy serum anti-D must be given if the patient's blood type is rhesus negative. A nursing care plan should be devised to include any additional discharge criteria. Figure 7.1 shows a specimen form used to ensure the application of agreed discharge criteria.

The nurse must ensure that the patient is accompanied home by a responsible adult and that suitable transport is available. This excludes being a pillion passenger on a motor bike, or the patient driving a car, or even a bus as has been known to happen. Although such a depth of questioning may seem unnecessary it is

DISCHARGE CRITERIA

	Yes	No	N/A		Yes	No	N/A
Do you have someone at home				Stable vital signs			
Responsible relative/friend to collect				Alert and Orientated			
TTO Drugs given/Check allergies				Diet and fluids taken			
Out Patient Appointment given				Pain/Nausea Controlled			
Sick certificate given				Bowels/Voided urine			
Valuables returned				Pack/Redivac removed			
Written and verbal discharge instructions given and agreed				Wound checked			
D. Nurse/Appointment for sutures				Dressing changed/Supply dressings given			
Questionnaire given				Venflon removed			
G.P. Letter given/faxed				Seen by Doctor			
Carer leaflet				Drug information leaflet/Pain killers			
Confirm Homecheck Number				Drug information leaflet/Antibiotics			

Signature_____ Date_____

Fig. 7.1 A specimen form used to ensure the application of agreed discharge criteria.

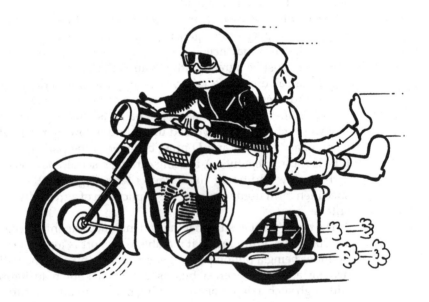

often found to be essential. Accompanying relatives/friends must come to the day unit and collect the patient. Patients have been known to inform the nurse they are meeting their escort outside the unit, but this is not acceptable because, once discharged, patients are keen to leave and have been known to walk home, baggage and all. One must also confirm that the relatives or friends will stay with the patient for the first night at home and that they understand and are confident about their duties as a carer.

Discharge criteria

Stable vital signs

The times when post-operative recordings of blood pressure and pulse rate are taken must be left to the discretion of the patient's nurse. The frequency of these recordings depends upon the patient's condition and any clinical signs which could indicate complications, for example chest pain, pallor, fainting and irritability. Nurses must always be fully aware that complications do occur following day surgery and any which arise must be identified quickly and treated, and special recordings may be requested following certain procedures, such as an arteriogram. The blood pressure and pulse rate should not be grossly different from the initial recordings taken at pre-assessment or admission to the day care unit even though these readings were taken when the patient was anxious and so might not represent a true normal for the patient. When blood pressure and pulse rate are abnormal it may be possible to compare them with a previous admission record, but if the nurse is in the least concerned guidance should be sought from medical staff. When discharging patients from the day surgery unit it is always advisable to err on the side of caution.

There should be no evidence of upper airway obstruction. Patients who are asthmatic or have other pre-existing respiratory problems must not leave the unit if their pre-anaesthetic status has worsened. Any signs of breathlessness, wheezing or stridor should be reported immediately to medical staff.

Alert and orientated

Before discharge patients must be alert. They should know where they are, the time of day and must be able to cooperate with and remember the discharge arrangements that have been agreed previously. For the majority of patients some sedative effect will remain from the use of anaesthetic drugs and analgesics. It is therefore the nurse's responsibility to ensure that when the patient is discharged they, and the person accompanying them, understand that they are still under the influence of mild sedation and that this will affect both memory and recall. Patients and carers should have this information readily available in the procedure-specific information leaflet and discharge leaflet.

If carers have been involved in the information process throughout the patient's progress through day surgery, they should be happy and confident to care for the patient on returning home. If they do voice concerns regarding the level of consciousness, the patient must be allowed a longer recovery time in the day unit and if insufficient time is available, as when the unit is closing, this patient must be transferred to an in-patient bed elsewhere.

Diet and fluids

On return from the first stage recovery area, oral fluids should be offered to the patient unless there are specific contraindications or nausea and vomiting occurs (experience has shown that the majority of patients will not accept fluids if feeling nauseated). Once oral fluids have been tolerated a light snack can be given. A call-order menu is required and the times when it is available should be pre-arranged with the hospital kitchen staff, and pre-packed sandwiches, toast, yogurts, fresh fruit and biscuits are the best kind of food to hold on the unit. Patients must be able to tolerate fluids and, preferably, a snack before discharge. Any specific diet instructions must be given and any restrictions in diet prior to surgery must either be continued or the patient informed these are no longer required.

Pain control

Patients must only be discharged from the day unit when the amount of pain or discomfort they are experiencing is acceptable to them. It is unrealistic to expect all patients to be totally pain free. Patients must be told if they have had local anaesthetic infiltrated into the wound because they will feel well and pain free when they leave the unit and may be overactive at home. In these cases, both the patient and relatives must be told that the local anaesthetic is blocking pain and that when pain starts analgesia is required promptly. Experience has shown that such patients require more support at home and contact the day unit by telephone more frequently.

It is good practice to give analgesia 30 to 60 minutes before discharge as this will allow the patient a comfortable journey home, though the need for this will differ with the speciality and is less dependent upon the procedure undertaken. When patients are in pain following any operation analgesia must not be withheld because pain thresholds vary greatly and it is inappropriate for the nurse to assess analgesia requirement on type or length of procedure.

Drug protocols are used by most day units, an example of which is shown in Fig. 7.2. Policies for the giving of drugs for patients to take home should be agreed by the clinicians and pharmacists and, for the majority of day surgery patients, pain can be well controlled with such a regime of oral analgesia.

Nausea

It is unacceptable for any patient to embark on a journey home while feeling nauseated or vomiting. Patients should only be discharged from the day unit when this has resolved. If necessary, arrangements should be made to transfer the patient to an in-patient bed. Antiemetics should always be given in conjunction with opiates and units should also consider issuing antiemetics as a routine to patients requiring strong analgesia at home. These need not be used if not required and it will prevent patients having to contact their GP for an antiemetic.

Voiding of urine

Unit policies vary relating to the voiding of urine before patients go home. There are those who require all patients to pass urine while others do not consider this necessary. Enforcing the former may cause an excessive stay for some patients and increase the risk of patient dissatisfaction. Patients kept nil orally for long periods will not be fully hydrated and may therefore not be able to pass urine on demand, so undue pressure from nursing staff

Post-operative pain treatment guidelines

Aim: To increase the awareness of pain control for junior hospital doctors, nursing staff and pharmacists. Pain care will be initiated in recovery. The aim is to discharge the patient home reasonably alert with their pain and nausea controlled. To improve the quality of care for all day/ short stay patients. These guidelines do not allow for atypical patients.

Type of pain	Analgesic	Dose ADULT ONLY	Side effects	Cautions Contra-indications
Mild to Moderate	Paracetamol	0.5g to 1.0g 4–6 hours Max 4g daily	Rash, blood disorders, acute pancreatitis, liver damage.	Hepatic and renal impairment, alcohol dependence.
Severe	Paracetamol 500mg with codeine 30mg	Day 1 Two every six hours Regularly not PRN. Day 2 Two every eight hours.	Dizziness, sedation, nausea, constipation.	Hepatic and renal impairment.
Excruciating	Pethidine sc or im	50mg to 100mg every 2–3 hours	Nausea and vomiting, sedation, constipation, respiratory depression, convulsions.	Head injuries, hepatic and renal impairment, asthma.

Nausea and vomiting

If codeine or pethidine is given, patients should be given an antiemetic drug to take out. Metoclopramide 10mgs TDS or prochlorperazine 5mgs TDS orally, intramuscular for inpatients.

Because of the side effects of antiemetics, they require limited prescription with reassessment.

Fig. 7.2   Staff advice on pain relief in the day surgery suite.

will increase pain and result in an over-anxious patient who is unable to produce urine. That said, the nurse must prevent complications occurring when the patient goes home and patients who have any predisposing condition which may lead to difficulty in voiding urine post-operatively will require special assessment, for example patients with prostate problems.

There are certain accepted high risk procedures where patients must void urine before leaving the unit, such as repair of inguinal hernia and some urological and gynaecological procedures. If the nurse has any concerns the urinary bladder size should be examined and, where necessary, medical staff should be informed of the difficulty.

Mobility

All patients must be able to move about alone without feeling faint or dizzy before they leave the unit. The activity must be consistent with their admission mobility and the procedure undertaken. All patients who have had an epidural or spinal anaesthetic must stand only when strength and sensation have returned, because any attempt to rush these patients could prove dangerous. Patients who are discharged following regional blocks in the hand and arm must be given full explanations regarding the length of time they will be without muscle power to prevent them falling or straining joints. Also, without the help of sensation, tissue damage from pressure or temperature change is a potential danger until mobility and sensation of the affected limb returns.

There are exceptions to the rule that all patients must return to full mobility before leaving the day unit, and these include patients who have undergone surgery to the lower limbs. Where patients are required to use crutches or a wheelchair at home, the nurse must ensure that they are seen by a physiotherapist and the first visit of the physiotherapist should preferably take place prior to the patient undergoing surgery. This enables patients to become familiar with the equipment they will use and they can show competency with these aids before leaving the unit. Where crutches are to be used patients should, if necessary, be shown how to go up and down stairs. It is essential for the day unit staff to cooperate with the physiotherapy department staff who must be convinced of the need and importance of pre-operative visits and after-care being completed in one day. To ensure that physiotherapy staff are available when required they should be informed of all orthopaedic admissions and any other physio-therapy requirements in the day unit one week in advance.

Surgical wound and dressings

Every surgical wound and/or dressing must be examined before the patient leaves the day unit and this should be part of every unit's discharge criteria. There must be no obvious bleeding or distension around the wound site. The dressing should be clean and dry, and if bleeding had been noted post-surgery (this will have been marked on the dressing and recorded on the nursing care plan), there should be no further extension of bleeding on the dressing. If there is bleeding this dressing must be removed and the wound site checked.

Following abdominal surgery the nurse must watch for any increase in girth or swelling and report this. Following gynae-cological surgery blood loss per vagina must be checked and any increase in volume and passing of blood clots noted. Anything unusual must be reported to medical staff. Following urological procedures the degree of haematuria should be noted.

All patients must have written information available which explains what should be expected after individual procedures and if a patient has any worries or concerns on returning home they must be encouraged to telephone the day unit. Even if calls seem unnecessary they should be graciously answered as they arise from anxiety.

Certain procedures include the insertion of a surgical drain. Providing drainage is minimal medical staff may request these to be removed, though some patients are discharged home with drains left in. Patients and carers must be informed about care of the drain while at home, and arrangements should be made for removal by community nursing staff or in the day unit.

Patients discharged from the day unit who require a change of dressing must be given a supply of these to take home with them and before they leave the unit the nurse must ensure that the dressing is comfortable and is in no way restrictive.

Those patients whose surgery necessitated the application of a plaster cast must be given written instructions covering the immediate 24 hours and general care. Before the patient leaves the unit the nurse must ensure that the encased limb is warm and well perfused and that the patient has normal sensation. Where indicated the provision of a sling for elevation of a limb may be required, and patients must be informed of when and for how long they are required to use the sling.

Insertion and removal of venous cannulae must be documented in the nursing care plan and a final check that these have been removed should be included as part of the discharge criteria.

Any specific instructions which are in addition to the procedure-specific information available in print, must be produced in written form for the patient.

Responsible care at home

As part of pre-assessment all patients having a general anaesthetic will have confirmed that they were able to make arrangements for transport home with an accompanying relative or friend. They will also have confirmed that this person will remain with them for the first 24 hours. On admission the nurse will have confirmed that these arrangements hold firm and that home circumstances have not changed.

Clear written discharge advice is essential to ensure patients understand the importance of care at home. Many patients misjudge their fitness post-operatively, while others refuse to accept the advice and support offered. Such patients often leave the day surgery nurse with problems that cannot be resolved and arrangements must be made to transfer these patients to an inpatient ward.

The nurse must beware of the patient who is expecting to return home and function in their pre-operative manner. The single parent and the mother with small children, for example, may not be able to cope with caring for the family as well as themselves. If these problems were not identified at pre-assessment it is the discharge nurse's responsibility to make every attempt to resolve the problem and, indeed, this highlights once again the need for detailed written information and meticulous pre-assessment.

The patient's carer must be given every opportunity to voice concerns and discuss any pre-conceived dangers. The nurse has the responsibility to allay any anxieties or fears because, if this is not achieved, both patient and carer will experience undue stress, resulting in more calls to the day unit and the GP, along with increased patient dissatisfaction. Patients and carers must be given the telephone number of the day unit with details of their named nurse attached, and wherever possible this nurse should deal with any enquiries from the assigned patient.

When paediatric patients are travelling in private transport a parent or carer must not act as driver, so two people are needed to take the child home.

Appointments

On leaving, patients should be given any necessary out-patient appointments. This may not always be possible for various reasons, for example if further investigations are required before the patient can be referred to out-patients. However the patient is more likely to receive the right treatment if there are formal arrangements for a future out-patients' appointment to be made later and the appropriate nurse/clinician to be informed. Clerical staff should be informed of any necessary appointments as soon as patients return from the operating theatre to allow time for these to be made. It is useful to designate this responsibility to one member of the clerical staff and ensure all nursing staff know of this arrangement.

Many patients are in full-time employment and to prevent an unnecessary visit to their GP, sickness certificates should be issued by the day unit nursing staff.

Return of valuables

Despite advice to the contrary patients often arrive in the day unit with valuables. Unbelievable though it may seem patients also leave the unit without asking for them to be returned. The nurse must check for valuables that have been placed in safe-keeping and return them to the patient.

Medication

Any medicines prescribed by medical staff must be obtained for the patient, and any written information on side effects and general information about the drugs should be available for the patient to take home. The list of drugs given to patients to take home is not vast and day units should maintain adequate stocks of these to avoid unnecessary delays while getting prescriptions from the pharmacy.

The nurse must ensure that patients have a supply of the drugs they normally take at home and see that these have not been cancelled. It is surprising the number of patients who volunteer information as they are about to leave to the effect that they have 'run out' of their normal medicines, in which case these should be provided.

Before any medicines are given to patients the nurse must always check that the patient has no known allergies. If allergies exist these must be checked against medicines given to take home. Any contraindication must be double-checked and medical staff informed.

GP letters

Every patient leaving the day unit will have a discharge letter from the hospital which they or their carer must deliver to the patient's GP surgery within 24 hours. The nurse must explain this is necessary to inform the doctor that their operation has been done and they have been discharged home. When patients understand the importance of this letter few are undelivered, though there is always a small group of patients who do not get this letter delivered and in some units it is practice for a second letter to be sent by post.

Day units may like to consider the use of a fax machine for this purpose as most GP surgeries have fax machines installed. Doctors and nurses are then assured of good communication which results in general satisfaction. If a doctor or nurse is called to see a patient at home they will then have all the relevant information to hand.

After-care arrangements

Patients must be told about arrangements made for the district nursing services to call at their home to change dressings or remove sutures and wherever possible these arrangements should be made at their GP surgery with the practice nurse. The patient will be given a letter for the attending nurse which explains the type of suture used and, where staples have been used, the instrument for removing these must be supplied.

Community nursing staff have limited supplies of dressings and equipment so it is the day surgery nurse's responsibility to arrange for the patient to take these home.

Written and verbal after-care instructions

All patients must be in possession of written discharge instructions like those shown in Fig. 7.3. The nurse must be sure that all necessary information required by the patient is included and that any specific additional information has been added. When both parties are in agreement the nurse and patient should sign this document.

Discharge by doctor/nurse

A record must be kept of who discharged the patient from the day unit (this will be a nurse or a doctor) and where a patient is not happy to leave the unit without seeing a member of the medical team, such a meeting must be arranged. When medical staff are busy elsewhere the patient should be told that this may lead to a delay in discharge time, though they should be encouraged to wait so that their request can be met. The nurse must remain supportive and sympathetic and not infer that the delay is entirely the patient's fault. It is worth remembering that a nurse having responsibility for discharge is a relatively new concept and some patients still expect to see a doctor before they leave the day unit.

Quality assurance

The use of a patient questionnaire to assess quality of service is essential to any day unit (see Chapter 9). These questionnaires are given to patients as they leave the unit and the nurse should explain the importance of returning them within a specified time. Patients must be convinced that their comments and suggestions will be taken seriously and it is always useful to inform patients of changes in the service that have been implemented by patients' views of the service. A prepaid envelope must be supplied.

Psychological care

By ensuring that all the discharge criteria have been agreed and met, nurses can be assured that all physical aspects of the patient's care have been addressed. However, the importance of psychological and emotional care should not be forgotten. Patients must never feel that the only priority of the nurse in the day surgery setting is to ascertain 'how many and how quickly' patients can be processed. With the pressures on day surgery units to perform more operations and treat more patients it is all too easy for the patient as a person to be neglected. The patient must never feel rushed, as to do this will lower the overall quality of care as perceived by the patient.

Many patients fear talking under the effects of anaesthesia while many others have dreams. These symptoms are quite often induced by the use of some anaesthetic drugs and this should be explained to the patient. Allowing patients time to discuss fears and anxieties usually resolves these problems.

Failure to meet discharge criteria

Unfortunately there will always be a small percentage of patients who do not meet the discharge criteria and require admission to an in-patient bed. There are many different reasons for this and the following are examples:

- the surgery undertaken was more extensive than planned
- pain and nausea
- lack of mobility
- dehydration due to hyperemesis
- complications following surgery or anaesthesia.

Patients requiring admission will be anxious regarding their condition and may also feel 'a nuisance' for not recovering as planned. Nursing staff must give a full explanation as to the cause of the problem and reassure patients that this does occasionally happen. The patient's relatives or friends should be informed that discharge will be delayed and, where known, a new discharge date should be given to allow relatives to make new arrangements. Relatives and friends may greet such transfers with a sigh of relief as they may have had serious doubts as to their own capabilities. The patient, however, will find this period of their

We do hope your stay with us has met your expectations.

The following is a list of discharge arrangements made by your Nurse and agreed with you. If you disagree with any of the information given, or require additional help, please discuss this with your Nurse, <u>before</u> leaving the Hospital.

YOUR DISCHARGE INFORMATION

Name of Consultant _____

Operation/Procedure performed

_____

Named of GP _____

Your named Nurse _____

Day/Short Stay Services

Day Surgery Contact Telephone Number

Direct Line _____

Date of discharge _____

You have been given the following Tablets/Medicines _____

_____

_____

_____

Please take painkillers regularly for 48 hours.

It is suggested you refrain from work for:-

_____ days _____ weeks

Responsible adult to collect _____

Responsible adult at home for first 24
hours _____

Do not drive, operate machinery or drink
alcohol for 24 hours following discharge.
Your reflexes and judgement are affected
by anaesthetic drugs.

You have a written information sheet and
understand the contents   YES/NO/NA

Questionnaire given/understood _____

To help us we would be grateful if you
would complete and return within 30 days
of discharge in the pre-paid envelope.

An Out Patient appointment has/has not
been made

on _____ time _____

Sick Certificate given   YES/NO

Your discharge letter is to be handed in to
your GP's surgery within 24 hours of
discharge. Please ask a relative/friend to do
this for you.

GP letter given/faxed   YES/NO

Your Nurse will contact you
at home by phone on _____

Contact phone No. confirmed   YES/NO

If you do not have a telephone, will a friend/
relative please phone the suite?   YES/NO

Patient to phone Day Surgery
Suite telephone No. _____

An appointment has been made at your
GP's surgery for removal of your stitches

Date _____ Time _____

Please make an appointment with your
GP's surgery on the above date for removal
of your stitches/dressing.

The District Nurse will call to attend to your
dressing/remove stitches

Date _____ Time _____

Additional information requested and
given

_____

_____

_____

_____

_____

_____

Nurse signature _____

Patient signature _____

Fig. 7.3 (above and opposite)   A discharge information leaflet for patients.

care very worrying and nursing staff need to be sympathetic and patient.

Upon transfer the day surgery nurse must send all the records held by the day surgery unit to the relevant hospital ward as the final discharge of this patient is now the responsibility of another area. All discharge planning available must be given to the accepting nurse.

There are day units now associated with 'patient hotels'. Where patients are fit for discharge but home circumstances are unsatisfactory, patients can be transferred to the hotel rather than an acute in-patient bed. Most hotels do not use qualified nursing staff, but they do allow patients to be treated who would otherwise be excluded from day surgery at pre-assessment because of unsatisfactory social circumstances.

Patient self discharge

There are occasions when patients demand discharge prematurely without prior agreement with medical staff. In these circumstances, the hospital policy on patients acting against advice applies to the day surgery setting and must be strictly followed. Wherever possible the nurse, medical staff and relatives must be involved in trying to persuade the patient to remain in the day unit until he or she is fit to be discharged, though in most instances this is to little avail as the patient is usually very determined to leave.

At this point the nurse must determine whether the patient meets agreed discharge criteria and, if they do not, the reasons must be carefully documented. Diplomacy and tact are required when dealing with these patients and it is imperative that the nurse behaves professionally and remains in control of the situation. The nurse should not deliberately attempt to delay discharge by whatever means. Patients have a legal right to discharge themselves.

Medical staff must always be informed of a patient's intention to self discharge and, when all else has failed, must explain to the patient they are taking their own discharge against medical advice. The patient should be requested to sign the appropriate form. If necessary the patient's GP must be contacted and the situation explained. Nursing records should be concise and accurate as to the course of events leading up to and during the patient's self discharge.

Key messages

    (1) Day care requires a method of ensuring fitness and proper home care after a procedure for all patients.

    (2) Planning from first patient contact is to enable patients to be self sufficient but not at risk.

    (3) The nurse discharge criteria must be precise, easy to apply and inviolable.

    (4) Written information is essential to minimise after-care anxiety and must include clear arrangements should an emergency arise.

References and further reading

Bradshaw, E.G. and Davenport, H.T. *Day Care – Surgery, Anaesthesia and Management*, Edward Arnold, London, 1989.

Jarrett, P.E.M. 'The pros and cons of day surgery', *Medical Monitor* 23, 15 (November, 1990).

Mortensen, M. and McMullin C. 'Discharge score for surgical outpatients', *American Journal of Nursing*, 86, 12 (1986), 1317–19.

Moscovici, S. *Social Influence and Social Change*, Academic Press, London, 1976.

Ogg, T. 'An assessment of post-operative outpatient cases', *British Medical Journal*, 4 (1972), 573–6.

Ruckley, C.V. *et al.* 'The community nurse and day surgery', *Nursing Times*, 76, 6 (February, 1980), 255–6.

Schneider, M. 'Criteria for discharge', in: Frost, E. (ed) *Recovery Room Practice*, Blackwell Science Inc., Boston, 1985.

Stephenson, M.E. 'Discharge criteria in day surgery', *Journal of Advanced Nursing*, 5 (1990), 601–13.

Chapter 8

Post-operative Pain, Nausea and Vomiting in the Day Surgery Patient

Susan Carrington

Introduction

Increasingly more advanced techniques are available on a day case basis for medical and surgical care with less after-effects. These developments have shifted the emphasis on how patient care is given by both hospital and community health staff so that patients and carers can take on a greater responsibility and participate more in how patient care is managed.

In the management of day surgery there need to be new priorities in order to achieve overall successful patient outcomes. These include:

- an exacting patient selection
- the absence of pain or nausea and vomiting in an alert post-operative patient who is discharged into the care of a responsible adult.

In 1993 a national survey of post-operative analgesia and control of emesis was undertaken in 231 day surgery units in England and Wales. The results indicate that nearly 70% of these units reported a problem with the management of pain in their units and 44% reported a problem with post-operative nausea and vomiting. The high incidence of these distressing post-operative complications in day surgery points to the importance of determining how they are managed.

Pain is addressed separately from nausea and vomiting although there are many similarities, both in prevention and treatment.

Factors influencing pain management

An underlying principle in pain management is that prevention is better than treatment. Once sensory input from injured tissues reaches spinal cord neurones the subsequent response is enhanced. Pain receptors in the periphery also become more sensitive, and so once pain is established there is a far greater problem than if it had been prevented or minimised in the first place.

Many studies show that acute pain is the result of inefficient treatment. The reasons for this are many. Principally it results from deficient knowledge or skill of health care staff and/or patients and their relatives.

We now know that different people may require very different levels of analgesia. Patients of the same age and sex having the same operation will have very different pain experiences, yet historically treatment regimes have been routine. One reason for patients' different experiences could be the different levels of endogenous opioids (that is the natural analgesics produced by each person's body). Simplistically a greater release of endogenous opioids may reduce the amount of analgesic drug required.

Psychological factors

Psychological factors can, and often do, play an important role in exacerbating or diminishing any individual's pain experience. They may include the degree of fear or anxiety a patient experiences during the whole day surgery visit, or they might be associated with the pain itself. Individuals have quite different coping strategies, life experiences and expectations and fears which modify pain appreciation.

Coping strategies

The locus or degree of pain control that people desire often indicates their coping strategy. Those patients with internal coping strategies (i.e. those who need to be in control of what is happening to them) will have a significant desire for detail about what is going to happen to them in order to cope with the situation. Patients who use external coping strategies (i.e. those who are dependent on the direction of others) block off information in order to cope. They come into hospital and are prepared to 'be done unto', and they do not wish to be given unsolicited details.

There can be different degrees of coping evident in people of different ethnic cultures, for instance some cultures favour the 'stiff upper lip' approach, while others are more ready to openly express their pain and feelings.

Life experiences

Patients with significant life experiences, such as severe emotional trauma or pain – divorce, loss of job, giving birth, previous surgery – may cope well with post-operative pain because they know it will pass and current pain may be less acute than before. Alternatively, people with chronic illness or pain may well enjoy the helplessness of dependence.

The extrovert type of personality may respond differently to the introvert. Extroverts may be able to describe their pain and clearly state what they want, while introverts may not be able to express themselves well and might find it more difficult to gain attention. However, they may have a tendency towards dependency and passively voice their needs.

Expectations and fears

Patients' fears and expectations can affect the degree of pain they suffer. For example, a patient donating an organ usually experiences less pain than the organ recipient who has the added fear of organ rejection and the very serious consequences of this.

Patient preparation

When preparing patients for any surgery, it is vital to give good clear advice which involves them in planning the management of their own pain. This principle is true for all, but there are two stipulations that need to be considered. One is that it is usually appropriate only to give as much detail as patients want, and the second is that having advocated patient involvement pre-operatively, it is crucial to follow that through. It would not be appropriate to start by encouraging patient involvement and then to remove their control and participation.

Care planning

Pre-admission

Information about pain control should start in the community. General practitioners and district nurses should be informed about techniques usually used in day surgery and the analgesic options available.

The subject of pain and pain control should be discussed at the out-patient and pre-admission interviews where the patient's main carer will hopefully be present. When the day surgery care is planned a full history of the patient's past pain experience is taken. The interviewer aims to find out about the patient and their family, to build a relationship of trust and to alleviate fear. Patients and their carers need the reassurance pre-operatively that discharge home will only occur when pain is controlled.

There are pre-operative pain assessment questionnaires available that will give a psychological profile of the patient, but simple questioning should suffice for a post-operative pain management plan in day surgery.

The planning of anaesthesia should take pain prevention into account.

On admission

It is crucial in the short pre-admission period that the nurse sits down and talks through with the patient how their pain will be managed. This includes information about the type of pain their operation can cause and details of how it can be relieved. By discussing options, like injections, prior to surgery, patients are better prepared for the likely outcomes. By having prior knowledge of what is available or the severity of the pain they may experience, patients are in a better position to make choices, though they will still require guidance at the time.

Treatment options available

There are three cornerstones to post-operative pain management in day surgery.

(1) The use of intravenous, opioid analgesics before, during or after surgery.
(2) The use of local anaesthetics for the operation, alone or as adjuncts to general anaesthesia and at the end of surgery.
(3) The use of oral analgesics and/or anti-inflammatory agents, both in the unit and on discharge.

Intramuscular opioids given post-operatively are not favourable because of the inevitable delay in their absorption into the bloodstream. This sometimes allows pain to become severe before the drugs can take effect. Intramuscular drugs can also have a depot (storage) effect, with a potentially delayed adverse reaction. Consequently, most day surgery patients will have an intravenous access route in recovery and an anaesthetist on site to give a first dose. In order to facilitate speedy management of post-operative pain the prescription should be available in the recovery room so that treatment of pain is given as soon as the patient experiences it. It could sometimes be the case that stronger analgesia is initially withheld because of concern on behalf of the carer that the patient may not be suitable for discharge that day and would need overnight admittance. However, once pain has become established it is much more difficult to control, will require larger doses of analgesia and leads to anxious patients and nurses. Furthermore, complications are likely to develop such as nausea and vomiting from the pain as well as increased side effects from the narcotics.

Local anaesthesia has a paramount role in day surgery post-operative pain control. This includes infiltration into wounds, regional blocks or topical application.

Oral analgesia

Oral drugs are given as the first option of pain control for minor surgery and they are also given in conjunction with local anaesthesia or after intravenous narcotic pain control.

As with intramuscular drug administration, it is important to recognise that an oral route takes time to be effective and the gut function can greatly influence the efficiency of entry to the blood. Non-steroidal anti-inflammatory drugs (NSAIDs) are well absorbed, relatively quick acting, and offer a potent analgesic effect. However, it is essential to be aware of contraindications to the use of NSAIDs. Contraindications are in the main gastro-intestinal bleeding, renal impairment or asthma.

Pain management protocol

A simple pain management protocol for day surgery is essential in planning individual patient's care. This could take the form of a flow chart or algorithm (see Fig. 8.1). Such plans are widely used on general surgical wards with the introduction of intravenous patient-controlled analgesia, epidurals, and acute pain management teams.

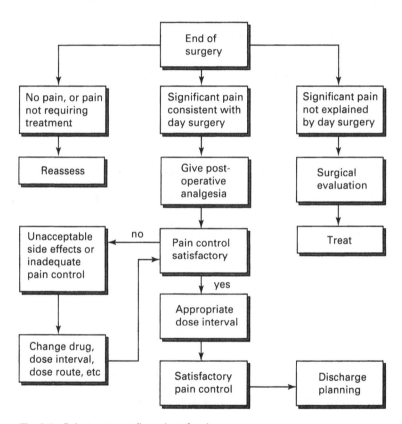

Fig. 8.1 Pain treatment flow chart for day surgery.

Monitoring pain

The initial relationship established between nurse and patient prior to admission will set the scene for how pain is both monitored and subsequently dealt with. Prior to surgery the pre-admission nurse stresses the importance of the patient letting the staff know when they have pain and how that amount of pain is monitored may vary. A visual or verbal analogue scale can be used (see the examples of pain intensity scales in Fig. 8.2) and if so, patients should be shown how to use them before surgery when planning their care. If this happens they will not then be upset during recovery by the questions when regular pain assessment is added to the monitoring of their vital functions.

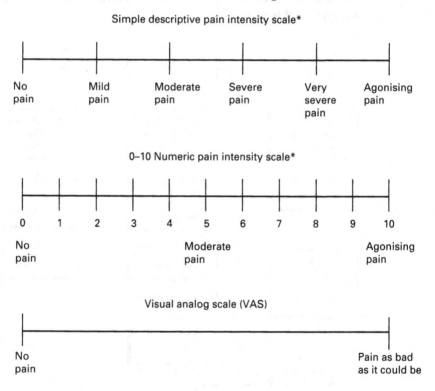

* If used as a graphic rating scale employ a 10 cm baseline

Fig. 8.2 Examples of pain intensity and pain distress scales.

In a day surgery unit the concept of patient-controlled analgesia can come into its own with patients and their relatives understanding the language and methods of pain assessment. Once anaesthesia has worn off, they can take control effectively of both their own pain assessment and subsequent relief. This may include explanation which reassures patients that they need not be frightened to move, or relaxation techniques and self medication.

It is important to advise patients to take their pain relief regularly to ensure a steady level of pain control and the same assessment tool should be used through to discharge. Advice should be given on discharge about what is a usual amount of pain to experience and what is excessive. Patients should also be advised of the warning signs to look out for and how to get help and reassurance should there be any concerns.

Paediatric post-operative pain

Management of post-operative pain in children is often even less satisfactory than in adults and its objective must be to offer the child the reassurance that they will experience no pain or minimal pain. Again prevention is better than cure.

Pain assessment in small children represents a real challenge. The way in which children give meaning to their pain and communicate that experience is dependent on their mental age and, as with adults, there are many influencing factors including their emotional state, family issues and attitudes, culture and environment. However, the management of a child's post-operative pain is made difficult because, unlike adults, infants and young children may not understand the reason for surgery or investigation. They may not participate actively in providing consent and young children cannot comprehend that some procedures must be done very quickly.

A pain history obtained prior to or at admission will focus on the language the child uses to describe his pain, for instance 'ow', 'ouch' or 'hurt'. This history may include family involvement in previous pain experiences, family coping strategies and the appropriate method of communication.

Caring for the child requires frequent assessment and reassessment of the presence, amount, quality and location of pain. It also means preventing or reducing anticipated pain and, when that is not possible, promptly alleviating pain.

The nurse, child and family can then decide together on their approach to pain assessment and treatment, and from pre-assessment onwards routine assessment and documentation of pain assessment is needed.

Treatment

There have been considerable anaesthetic advances in paediatric day surgery pain management, most notably the use of local anaesthetic techniques, NSAIDs and EMLA cream.

Pain is managed by the child, parent and their carers, and effective interaction is vital. Whenever possible through the day parents or a nurse should be with the child because a sense of security is the source of great comfort. The parents' knowledge of the child is invaluable for patient and day surgery staff, though parents must be given the necessary information before the day so that they know what to do, where to be and what to say to help the child. While it is important to respect the child's wishes, the nurse's first priority has to be the safety of the patient.

As with adults, children's pain must be controlled before they go home. The named nurse must ensure that the child's carers know what to look for, what is normal, how to safely administer analgesia, what to do if it is inadequate, and how to get help and advice if needed. In the past it was taught that narcotic analgesics should be avoided particularly with children because of the risks of side effects and because assessment of efficiency is difficult. There is less fear of side effects now, and current wisdom holds it better for babies to be relieved from their pain than to suffer it. Nevertheless, analgesics must be administered very carefully to babies.

Post-operative nausea and vomiting (PONV)

Most nausea and vomiting is not significantly life threatening, but it is an enormously distressing and frightening experience. Severe persistent vomiting can have very serious results, including death.

The situation is more easily handled in in-patients where sedative side effects of antiemetics are not a problem. In day surgery, either this post-operative complication or its subsequent treatment can greatly delay discharge times or lead to unanticipated hospital admission.

Stress must be placed upon a prophylactic approach to post-operative nausea and vomiting rather than a therapeutic one. The first step is to identify patients of high risk so that preventative steps can minimise the incidence.

Patients who have experienced post-operative nausea and

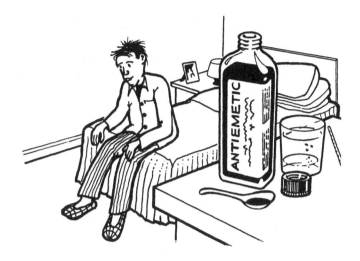

vomiting in the past are often extremely anxious about the prospect of a repeat experience. This in turn can exacerbate the situation.

Pre-operative care planning

It is vital during pre-operative assessment to gather information from the patient and their relatives that will give some indication of susceptibility to PONV and suggest the best subsequent treatment. The following predisposing factors should be ascertained.

(1) A history of nausea and vomiting following general anaesthesia – this could, for example be provoked by hospital smells and sounds.
(2) Age and weight – those aged from three to thirteen and anyone suffering from obesity are most at risk.
(3) The female gender – women suffer more from PONV than men, especially in relation to menstruation.
(4) A history of motion sickness or migraine – most relevant when rapid mobilisation is intended.
(5) A familial history of post-operative nausea and vomiting.
(6) Surgery – some operations, such as laparoscopic gynaecology, take a long time and require fluid restriction before,

during and after the procedure, all of which make PONV more likely.

(7) A full stomach through unabsorbed ingested food or through pathology.

(8) Anaesthetics are now less emetogenic, but with excess depth or duration of anaesthesia gut distension or hypotension can increase post-operative nausea and vomiting, as can complementary opioid administration.

Therapy

The presentation of any combination of predisposing factors would indicate the use of preventative therapy. Then an antienitic regime is prescribed pre-operatively. After surgery, early identification of nausea and vomiting is important. Explanation and reassurance need to be given to patients about why they are experiencing these upsets and how this is to be managed. If treatment fails it will be necessary to combine drugs with different actions.

Delay in sitting up or mobilisation because of nausea can be frustrating to patients. Again they need treatment, reassurance and time. Having vomited or simply feeling unwell can be frightening for patients. They will feel a loss of control and loss of dignity, and may even feel that they are inconveniencing people with what is not a serious condition. Here again, a good relationship between nurse and patient is vital in order to offer care of very intimate needs.

A further challenge to the management of post-operative nausea and vomiting in a day surgery patient is the side effect of current drug therapy, particularly that of sedation. New treatments, although expensive, can be worthwhile if they mean a patient's distress can be minimised, and especially if they can avoid an overnight admission.

It must be recognised that there are some patients in whom it is extremely difficult to control sickness. Treatment in such cases needs to be aggressive. It is more appropriate to admit a sedated patient with controlled nausea and vomiting than one who is unsedated with uncontrolled nausea and vomiting. How such a situation is managed from the outset could mean the difference between a traumatic experience, and a carefully explained, understood course of events for patients and their carers.

Maintain fluid balance

Care should be taken to ensure that patients are told pre-operatively about the importance of hydration prior to surgery. Fluid intake should not be restricted until three hours before surgery unless contraindicated and instructed. Apart from maintaining pre-operative comfort by not depriving patients of fluids until necessary, dehydration would exacerbate post-operative nausea and vomiting. Conversely, before discharge from the day surgery unit it may be better to let patients decide whether or not they want to drink because enforced drinking may increase the incidence of nausea and vomiting.

Discharge

The importance of patient education is paramount when planning the safe discharge of patients. They and their carers need to be warned about the possibility of nausea and vomiting on discharge. A patient may be perfectly well in the day surgery unit, but the journey home could cause nausea or vomiting. Advice would include what to do, at what point to be alarmed and who to contact.

Key messages

(1) What may be considered early 'minor' post-operative complications in hospital are of more consequence for patients returning to and at home.

(2) The two commonest disruptive problems are pain and PONV. If they are likely to be very disruptive or are uncontrolled, they prohibit day care.

(3) The pain-conscious nurse will provide explanation, seek prevention and ensure structured treatment with minimally discomforted patients.

(4) Nurse identification of patients with a high risk of PONV possibly by check-list, will enable preventive measures and optimal antiemetic drug use.

References and further reading

Ellersen, E., Anderson, H.B., Eliasen *et al.* 'A comparison between pre-incisional and post-incisional lignocaine infiltration and post-operative pain', *Anaesth. Analg.* 1994; 495–498.

Hawthorn, J. *Understanding and Management of Nausea and Vomiting,* Blackwell Science Ltd, Oxford, 1995.

Leith, S.E., Hawkshaw, D. and Jackson, I.J.B. 'A national survey of the importance of drug treatment of pain and emesis following day surgery', *Journal of One-Day Surgery,* 4: 2 (1993), 24–5.

Ogg, T.W. and Hitchcock, M. 'Post-operative nausea and vomiting', *Journal of One-Day Surgery* 1994; 2; 18–19.

US Department of Health and Human Services. Clinical Practical Guideline – Acute Pain Management: Operative or Medical Procedures and Trauma, RCA Public Health Service. Agency for Health Care Policy and Research. Feb. 1992.

Chapter 9
Follow-up Arrangements
Moira Edmondson

Introduction

The safe discharge of all patients from the day surgery unit must be a prime objective but their care does not and must not finish there. Each patient admitted to the day unit has undergone a surgical procedure or investigation and been discharged home, all within a short space of time. Despite the high quality care and production of specific written information, patients still fear being at home without being able to have further contact with the day surgery unit nursing staff. The holistic approach to care used in day surgery means the nurse has a responsibility to ensure that contact is made with all patients at home following discharge. This contact must be considered an integral part of the day surgery patient's experience and one which they must have a right to expect from a caring profession.

'Homecheck' telephone calls, patient satisfaction surveys and quality review groups must become accepted practice in all day units if we are to maintain a safe and high quality service. This chapter discusses the follow-up arrangements which day units should consider as part of the service offered to day surgery patients.

'Homecheck'

Patients are informed when being discharged by their nurse that they will be contacted at home by telephone the day following surgery. There will be occasions when the nurse will need to refer patients to their GP, and it is essential that these calls are made by a qualified nurse who has the knowledge and experience to answer any questions and deal with all problems. It is also the day surgery nurse's responsibility, where appropriate, to invite the patient to reattend the day unit. Experience has shown that the number of patients requiring a return visit to the unit is very small, for example in a six-month period in Canterbury only four patients were requested to return out of 3500 patients treated. This results in little impact on nursing workload. Where referral to the patient's GP is required the nurse should contact the patient later that day to find out about any treatment given and ensure they have no further problems.

To ensure an efficient service is offered and privacy is maintained the nurse should confirm the following with the patient:

- a contact telephone number and whether this is different from their home telephone number
- any particular times contact would be inconvenient
- whether the nurse may or may not reveal their identity
- whether contact is only to be made with the patient (i.e. do not discuss with the patient's family).

It is essential that the nurse documents the date and time of this interview and it is useful to agree a contact time with patients and carers before they leave the unit. This time must wherever possible be adhered to. Early morning telephone calls are inappropriate as they could disturb both the patient and their family, but the interview should not be left until late in the day as this may leave patients with unresolved problems or untreated pain. There are occasions when, despite the agreement of a contact time, patients and carers are not available. A standard must be agreed within the unit as to the number of attempts at contact which can be made considering the daily workload and staffing levels within the unit. It is usually acceptable to make two attempts at contact and, where the patient is still unavailable, this must be documented. If the unit considers contact is mandatory, further attempts should be taken by nursing staff, when time permits, throughout the day.

Contact with patients should, wherever possible, be made by the patient's named nurse resulting in continuity of care for the patient and job satisfaction for the nurse. If the discharge nurse knows they will be unavailable at the time arranged for the telephone call, patients should be told the name of the nurse who will be contacting them. Where advice is given by the nurse, for example when pain has not been controlled, the patient should be informed that they will be contacted again later that day. A further contact time should be agreed for the patient's nurse to review the situation.

There may be occasions when patients decline the follow-up phone call, for example when they are undergoing termination of pregnancy. When this does occur the nurse should request that the patient contact the day unit at a mutually convenient time. In this way the right to privacy and confidentiality is respected and maintained at all times.

To facilitate the maintenance of accurate records of all home contacts, day units must design and implement the use of suitable documents in addition to their nursing notes. When completed these must be filed with the patients' records. An example of a 'homecheck' document is shown in Fig. 9.1.

Once 'homecheck' with internal audit is established consideration should be given to a further telephone call to the patient one to two weeks post-operatively. Patients' perception of their care and treatment can and does change once the effects of drugs and stress have resolved, particularly if complications have occurred. The same nursing 'homecheck' document should be used to enable a comparison of data which can then be used by the nursing team to implement change and improve the service.

The 'homecheck' service must be offered to all patients. Those patients who have undergone surgery under local anaesthesia must not be excluded on the grounds that it was 'only a minor procedure'. We have found that, when this group of patients was not contacted the following day, some of them can experience more problems than patients undergoing surgery with a general anaesthetic.

Those patients discharged on a Friday must be contacted the following day and not left until the following Monday. Not only is the day surgery unit closed but many GP surgeries only offer an emergency service on Saturday. This group of patients is consequently at great risk of becoming frightened, isolated and vulnerable, with minor problems becoming exaggerated. It is unrealistic for these patients to receive a telephone call from their named nurse as this would be an inefficient use of nursing resources. One nurse must be rostered each week to contact patients on a Saturday morning and experience has shown that the most suitable time for patients to receive this call is between 0900 hrs and 1100 hrs.

The telephone call

Interviewing patients by telephone demands patience and interviewing skills must be developed by the nurse. The initial

DAY SURGERY DIRECTORATE
HOME CHECK

Affix Patient Label:-

Home Telephone Number:-

Consultant:-

Date: Time:

Operation:-   GA/LA

Discharge Date:-

1.   Introduction (by Named Nurse)   YES/NO

2.   Problems encountered on journey home?   YES/NO
     a)
     b)

3.   Did you have a good night's sleep?   YES/NO

4.   Were you given painkillers?   In Hospital   YES/NO
                                   At Home   YES/NO
     Were you given painkillers to take home?   YES/NO

     Name of analgesia:-
     Tylex:-   Panadol:-   Other:-
     Codydramol:-   Voltarol:-

     Have you painkillers at home? If so, what:-

5. Is your pain controlled? If not, what level of pain is being experienced?
   State any advice given.

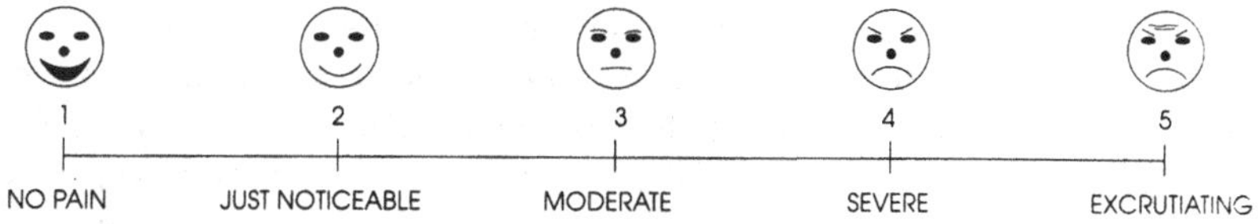

1	2	3	4	5
NO PAIN	JUST NOTICEABLE	MODERATE	SEVERE	EXCRUTIATING

6. Are there any specific problems relating to your surgery/wound etc?   YES/NO

   a)

   b)

7. Are there any specific problems relating to your care at home? YES/NO

   a)

   b)

8. Do you require any further advice?   YES/NO

   If yes, explain!

9. Does the patient need referral to:-

   GP   YES/NO   Distict Nurse?   YES/NO   Other?   YES/NO

   If YES, what advice given/action taken?

   _____

   _____

   _____

   _____

   _____

10. Confirm patient has telephone No. of ward and name of nurse to contact if any problems.

11. Any further advice/action taken. List below.

    a)

    b)

    c)

Signature of Nurse

Fig. 9.1 (above and opposite)   Day surgery directorate 'homecheck' document.

introduction should be warm and friendly, with the nurse speaking slowly and clearly. The patient must be made to feel that the nurse has time to talk and discuss any worries or problems. Questions, when asked, should not result in a plain 'yes' or 'no' answer and patients must be given the opportunity to describe how they feel or discuss any problems they have, in their own words and time. The temptation to complete a sentence for the patient should be resisted as it can result in the nurse missing vital information.

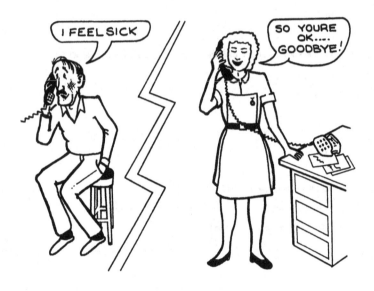

The 'homecheck' service does have financial implications. On average phone calls take three to four minutes for each patient, though there will always be the exception where more time is taken. Additional funding must therefore be obtained prior to commencement of this service. The changes in nursing establishment needed for follow-up of patients is dependent upon the activity of the unit. Weekly audit of 'homecheck' documents must be completed by the ward manager and correlation of this data can be used to identify any outstanding problems with particular groups of patients so that appropriate action/recommendations can be made. Following audit these forms should be filed in the patients' case notes.

Patient satisfaction survey

The service provided in the day unit should meet the requirements and demands of the local need. To ensure this need is being met, patient satisfaction surveys should be carried out at agreed intervals over a one-year period. These times will differ in individual units but it is essential that these surveys are undertaken at least once a year and ideally they should be carried out biannually over a three-month period, that is three months of survey will be followed by three months without survey. This gives staff the opportunity to correlate information and take corrective action.

Before approaching the task of writing a questionnaire the ward team must be clear about the usefulness of obtaining appropriate information. Units must have clear objectives because, all too often, poorly planned questionnaires are put together with every good intent by nursing staff. Subjective questions will be of no real value in determining the quality of the service and professional help should be sought in compiling the questionnaire.

Questionnaires are used to elicit specific information from patients to identify areas of dissatisfaction with the service provided, so any questions which cannot result in opportunities to make productive changes should be avoided. One area that must be included is the quality and content of the information received by patients. The professional's perception of the information required by patients is often distinctly different from that requested by patients and too often it is dictatorial in approach. Many exciting opportunities will present themselves to invoke change in style and quality of information leaflets by involving the patients in the compilation of their content.

Patients should be given questionnaires before leaving the unit, when the purpose and importance of completing these can be explained. A prepaid envelope should be provided and the patient requested to return the questionnaire within an agreed period of time, for example within 30 days. Allowing patients time to complete the questionnaire at home ensures the patient anonymity and privacy, and the effect of analgesic drugs and/or sedatives will be less likely later on. There is also a greater response rate with questionnaires when patients are given the opportunity to complete them at home in their own time. Experience has shown that where patients are expected to complete satisfaction surveys before leaving the unit they are often incomplete or not completed at all, partly because they are generally grateful for the care they have received and do not like to complain. We must ensure they do not feel pressurised by being indebted and that they know we genuinely need their honest comments.

As with all patient information the style and content of the questionnaire should be kept simple and a tick system for completion enables patients to answer questions easily. However, patients should be encouraged to write comments and ample space must be left between questions to permit this. It is useful to separate different aspects of the patients' care into sections and this also simplifies correlation. For example the following as group headings may be considered:

- pre-assessment
- the admission letter and information leaflet
- the admission day
- pain relief
- discharge information
- general questions.

In providing questionnaires patients who are not totally satisfied with their care are given the opportunity to voice their dissatisfaction.

In addition to the questionnaire, day surgery units may like to consider the forming of a quality review group, the purpose of which is described below (see also Chapter 10).

Quality assurance review group

It is essential that any patient expressing dissatisfaction in their survey is contacted and given the opportunity to discuss matters further. This can be achieved by asking all patients to write their name, address and telephone number on their questionnaire if they are willing to return to the unit to discuss the problems or difficulties they encountered before, during and after their stay. All such patients then receive a letter from the day surgery manager requesting they attend a quality review group meeting, which is best held outside working hours so that all those who work in the unit may attend. An agenda is published and sent to the patients attending and to representatives from the hospital Trust one week before the meeting. It is important that those representing the hospital Trust do not exceed the number of attending patients as this could be seen as a board of defence and would be intimidating for most patients. Representing the Trust, where possible, should be the chief executive and director of nursing and, from the day surgery unit, the director and manager. Depending on points raised on the agenda, wider representation from the Trust may be required, such as catering.

The meeting should be informal with light refreshments provided. One member of the Trust should chair the meeting and should allot time to each point on the agenda. Patients should be welcomed and thanked for attending the meeting and introduced to all those present. Where specific points raised cannot be answered and need further investigation this should be explained to the group. Wherever possible the meeting should last no longer than one hour, but each patient must be given the opportunity to voice their opinion. Occasionally patients wish to discuss problems in more depth privately and time must be allowed at the close of meeting for this to take place.

Before closing the meeting patients are informed that they will receive a copy of the minutes and notice of what changes will be made by the Trust to practice/procedures to improve the service. Following the close of such meetings patients generally enjoy a chat among themselves and with the staff present and often the last patient leaves at 2000 hrs. This must be considered when deciding dates for meetings and staff must be aware of the time commitment involved. It is bad to hurry patients off the premises when they have taken time to attend and this would certainly create a poor impression.

It would be fair to say that, following the initial decision to hold these meetings, a feeling of marked trepidation is apparent. Will there be verbal abuse? Will it result in a general moaning session? The answer to both of these questions is NO. We have found the criticism to be very constructive and many of the problems identified by patients simple to resolve. One word of caution, when involving day surgery staff in the group for experience there may be those who take patients' criticism personally. Such staff members can become very demoralised by the whole process and should not be forced to participate.

The following are examples of patient dissatisfaction and changes made at the Kent and Canterbury Hospitals Trust day surgery unit:

(a) **Problem: laparoscopic surgery**
  A large percentage of patients undergoing laparoscopic surgery complained of the discomfort experienced while

recovering on a trolley. Patients stated that they could not roll onto their side and draw their legs up to be comfortable.
Change
All patients undergoing laparoscopic surgery now recover on beds.
No further complaints received.

(b)   **Problem: mixes sex recovery areas**
Many patients objected to mixed sex recovery areas. This was particularly true for patients undergoing gynaecological procedures.
Change
All patients are now nursed in single sex bays.
In exceptional circumstances when we cannot fulfil this patients are offered an alternative date for admission.
No further complaints received.

(c)   **Problem: telephone messages**
Patients complained that they did not always receive telephone messages from relatives.
Change
Telephone message pads are now used by staff. These slips are adhesive and fixed to patients' lockers. This obviously helps when patients are still feeling drowsy.
No further complaints.

All problems raised by patients are discussed at the monthly unit meeting when all staff are involved in decisions made to change practice or procedures. The questionnaire is reviewed annually and amended accordingly using information obtained from previous correlations and to cover any new procedures or practice.

If information received from all the above quality initiatives is stored on a database this can be used to highlight specific trends in patients' comments. Changes made to improve the quality of care can then be monitored for their effectiveness and further action taken where necessary. This information should be made available to all areas within the Trust.

Contacting patients following discharge to evaluate the service is a nursing responsibility, as home circumstances may have changed and both carers and patients may require further advice and help. A further extension of that care worthy of consideration is whether a member of the day surgery team visits patients requiring assistance as dictated by the use of 'homecheck'. This holistic approach to patient care will lead to greater job satisfaction for the day surgery nurse who can then share in the success of the patient's full recovery.

Key messages

(1) Patient follow-up after day care is not a refinement but an integral part of the service.
(2) The better the follow-up the more the chance of improving the outcome at the time and for others in the future.
(3) A complete follow-up needs an investment of time and money with the intent of producing a 'patient marketeer' through patient satisfaction.

References and further reading

Audit Commission *A Short Cut to Better Services – Day Surgery in England and Wales*, HMSO, London, 1990.

Day Surgery Task Force *Day Surgery*, Department of Health, London, September 1993.

Garraway, W.M., Cuthbertson, C., Fenwick, N., Ruckley, C.V. and Prescott, R.J. 'Consumer acceptability of day care after operations for hernia or varicose veins', *Journal of Epidemiology and Community Health*, 32 (1978), 219–21.

Johnson, C.D. and Jarrett, P.E.M. 'Admission to hospital after day care surgery', *Annals of Royal College of Surgeons of England*, 72 (1990), 225–8.

Royal College of Surgeons of England *Guidelines for Day Care Surgery*, Royal College of Surgeons, London, 1992.

White, A.E. 'An evaluation of the paediatric home care scheme', *Journal of Advanced Nursing*, 16 (1991), 1413–21.

Young, C. 'The post-operative follow-up phone call: an essential part of the ambulatory nurse's job', *Journal of Post Anaesthesia Nursing*, 5 (1990), 273–5.

Chapter 10
Quality Assurance in Day Care

Susan Carrington

Introduction

Within the current health service market environment, there has been a shift from secondary to primary care. Part of this shift is the increase in day surgery activity, which is not a strategic goal in itself but a means of achieving many other strategic goals. These include the delivery of more appropriate care and better use of resources.

Further expansion and development of day surgery will be influenced strongly by customer attitudes, primarily those of patients but also their carers at home. In day surgery there is a comprehensive approach to patient care. The day surgery unit provides a service that starts before a patient arrives and extends after they are discharged. Care is given by members of a team who come from many disciplines and, in order to deliver care to patients, there is a need to support and develop the care givers.

A total quality system incorporates both of these aspects. That is, it supports and develops staff so that they can provide the optimum service to patients. It could be considered the two sides of a coin, one side patients, one side staff, thus involving both patients and staff in determining and evaluating how care is given.

Quality has always been the essential basis of professional health care standards. Total quality management (TQM) switches the focus from quality practised by professionals to the very organisation itself. The philosophy behind TQM was developed in the 1950s by the American business gurus William Deming and Joseph Juran and was pioneered in Japan. However, it was only in the late 1980s that the TQM philosophy of an organisation-wide meeting of customer needs was adopted by the British National Health Service.

A day surgery unit is usually a subsystem within a system – a unit within a hospital or Trust. So how can TQM be introduced into day surgery when it is only part of a much bigger organisation? The answer lies in the unique way that day surgery is organised. Unlike other departments in a hospital it can largely stand alone in the delivery of care and achievement of successful patient outcomes, and it is managed by a cohesive team. These two factors embody the principles of TQM.

To incorporate such beliefs and cultural change takes time. Initially, the quality plan seeks to establish standards of care and then gathers together indicators currently used to monitor the delivery of care, developing and expanding on these as awareness of such a process grows. It does not seek to reinvent the wheel, merely to offer a system of constant improvement. This chapter presents an outline of how to involve the day surgery team from the outset, including how to gain their commitment to establishing a system of total quality care and how to involve them in the entire decision-making process.

The groundwork

From the start there needs to be a clear understanding of the commitment you expect from people. Initial standards should be drawn up to ensure the highest possible quality care in a compassionate and cost effective way. Inherent in this is the use of the nursing assessment process which will include consideration of psychological, environmental, educational and discharge planning factors within a self-care model. Integral to this is the need to acknowledge that efficiency is a legitimate part of quality.

The objectives of the total quality plan will be to:

- support and develop the care givers, not only in what they do, but how it is done
- identify what standards should be set
- audit the processes of service delivery to the required standard, both in terms of efficiency and customer satisfaction
- identify appropriate performance indicators and measure these.

Cost

We now operate in a competitive environment and must therefore consider the cost of providing an efficient service.

Day surgery not only offers purchasers an effective form of treatment for less money, it also provides high quality care. It is the latter that will appeal greatly to customers of the future and it is widely believed that delivering a high quality service produces measurable benefits in profit, cost savings and market share. Day surgery is in a strong market position. This may represent a fairly radical change of attitude, but cost needs to form a clear basis to work from if we are to provide the service we would wish.

The quality team

The essence of a total quality plan is to encourage everyone to contribute their best, both as individuals and as members of a team, and to achieve this everyone must be involved from the outset.

There will inevitably be different personalities from different groups and/or professions. Because of this they will be motivated in different ways and have different priorities, which might include:

- better patient care
- being part of a team
- a happier place to work
- getting ahead
- cost efficiency
- a secure future.

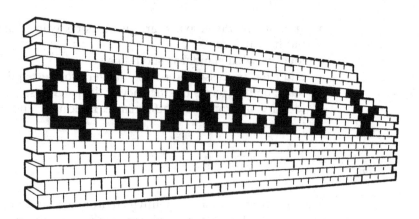

It is important to identify what the benefits are of developing a quality service for all concerned. However, if the plan is to succeed from the outset there needs to be commitment to the exercise from the top. There must also be a core team of people representing various groups as this will ensure a good cross-section of ideas and the widest possible dissemination of information. There is a temptation simply to include all the enthusiasts, but this is perhaps not the best strategy.

Within any group of people, specific personality types can be identified. The two key ones for a quality group are the two extremes of negative and positive individuals. The former would represent a strong voice against change. These individuals often have considerable experience, some of which may have resulted in their scepticism. However, they will have significant energy which, if directed, could significantly advance any venture. Also, although the initial reason for questioning any change or new idea may be doubt, that kind of scrutiny will often encourage attention to detail and proper planning on the part of the initiators. This will ensure projects are carefully thought through and discussed before being implemented.

The second group are the enthusiasts or strong positives, and they may need the control provided by non-enthusiasts. However, these enthusiasts are vital, particularly if they have excellent interpersonal skills, communication skills and perseverance, as they will help to move the planning forwards. With a fair balance of these two personality types, progress will be stimulated.

Previous quality initiatives

From the outset it is important to remember that a great deal of effort may already have been put into developing quality initiatives. These need to be built on and nurtured by giving people the latitude to develop their own methods as part of the plan. Recognising the importance of these can be strongly motivational.

Training

Crucial interpersonal training is needed for a team to grow. This will include team building, the management of change, influencing skills, customer care, self development and analysis of needs. Such training will improve communication and relationships within the unit. It will create a greater understanding of the differences in perception and interpretation of events and interchanges.

Rewards

Having established your team, the ultimate need is an in-built reward system. Individual performance appraisal will be a part of this, but perhaps the most important reward, and also the least costly, is praise. For example, it is helpful to organise quality events which offer the team recognition. This will not only publicly acknowledge the individual's or team's input and results, but will also encourage others.

The total quality plan aim is to get everyone in the unit working to achieve maximum efficiency. If we are to care for patients to the standard that we strive for, the unit needs to work well. If there are hitches and delays in the working of the unit, it is both patients and staff who suffer.

The key ingredient of teamwork is to encourage staff to take on a greater responsibility for their own work in order to fulfil a larger role in decision making. Such empowerment is based on the belief that people work better if they take part in decisions and that they know best how to improve their own job.

Patient involvement

The kernel of TQM has to be patient satisfaction, in the same way that businesses which remain successful focus on customer satisfaction. Look at how Ford cars have changed their approach to achieve this. Henry Ford's famous comment: 'You can have any colour you like so long as it's black' has been replaced by today's customer-oriented slogan: 'Everything we do is driven by you.'

The total quality plan means involving patients in planning services, reviewing the effectiveness of those services and, where possible, involving them in the actual process of care.

In the past, health care was very much planned by professionals and administrators who decided the needs of the patients. Although this was largely well intentioned, it did not necessarily suit the patients' actual needs. By auditing patients' desires we can develop new services and help close the gap between what patients expect and what we can provide. This in turn fosters an image of the quality and reliability of the service.

Studying customer satisfaction means much more than the occasional patient survey. It must be part of the overall plan, with specific auditing tools, including well-designed patient questionnaires suitable for the target audience. The easiest way to achieve this is to involve patients in devising the questionnaire. It is also vital to act on the information obtained from patients, again by involving them and all staff concerned.

The day surgery unit offers the newest opportunity to bring the appropriate resources and people together and to let them get on with it. In these units there is usually an in-built team spirit which involves everyone in the decision-making process. There needs to be a flexible and sensitive environment which seeks to find out what customers require and combines this with human resources (people) and tools and equipment (capital investment). It is then possible to produce a wide range of services which will give satisfaction.

The total quality plan provides a monitoring system which is run annually to allow a systematic measurement of the standard of care provided.

The total quality plan

The plan gathers together a wide range of indicators to assess the service delivered. Many of these may already be in use, some which are specifically designed for day surgery and others that require adaptation, depending on the specific area to be monitored. The indicators include:

- continuous quality improvement monitoring
- an assessment tool for the nursing care plan
- post-operative telephone calls
- patient satisfaction surveys
- staff development programme/monitoring tool
- hazard surveillance survey
- risk assessment.

Total quality leadership plan

Objectives

The objectives of the plan are to:

(1) Provide a systematic and ongoing process to monitor the quality and appropriateness of patient care.
(2) Seek opportunities to improve patient care and resolve identified problems.
(3) Continuously assess the quality and cost effectiveness of all products, services and information.
(4) Reduce risk in the clinical aspects of patient care and ensure visitor and employee safety.
(5) Ensure the appropriate and accepted professional standards of care are met.
(6) Involve the day surgery team in drawing up, implementing and evaluating the plan.
(7) Ensure effective communication systems, both within the unit and externally.
(8) Evaluate the effectiveness of the plan in its entirety, on a systematic basis.

Implementation

Assigning responsibility for the overall quality of care is of the utmost importance. The plan needs to be led from the top and the manager will delegate responsibility to others as they lead initiatives. Such responsibilities will incorporate and involve the direction and guidance of various clinical specialists.

The core team should be made up of representatives of all the different disciplines so that maximum input of ideas and dissemination of information can be achieved. The group will determine how aspects of care will be chosen for ongoing monitoring, they will provide feedback and incorporate improvements as planned.

There are certain key aspects of patient care that should be chosen as the most important to the quality of patient care and service provided. These should include, but not be limited to:

• nursing care
• patient information

- patient preparation for surgical procedures
- medical administration
- infection control
- maintenance of equipment and a safe environment
- audit of clinical outcomes.

How to monitor that the appropriate standard of care is being delivered

First, the day surgery team needs to determine the required standard of care. This can be achieved by the following means:

(1) A unit policy which clearly indicates the clinical guidelines for the selection of day surgery patients, and the subsequent discharge criteria for day surgery patients.

(2) Professional standards as determined by the unit staff, for example nursing standards referring to authoritative sources such as health care literature, research, clinical experts in their own disciplines, and their own experience. Having set these standards, the same professionals can determine what measures (indicators) would be most useful in monitoring those standards.

(3) Monitoring tools – indicators. These will vary in design, require regular modification according to need and they could include:
   - staff development programmes
   - patient satisfaction surveys
   - patient outcome variance reports
   - clinical outcome statistics
   - financial data analysis
   - assessment of nursing care plans
   - staff satisfaction surveys
   - risk assessments and hazard surveillance.

Actual monitoring of care

Having determined the standards to be achieved and the tools needed to monitor them, the next step is to plan how the monitoring processes will be set up. The goal is to gather enough information to be of value. Certain aspects will need to be concurrent, for example it is useful to monitor patient satisfaction while auditing nursing assessment so that any irregularities can be cross-referenced.

Some auditing will be continuous such as variance monitoring and it will be necessary to determine at what point to pick up that information. The easiest way is to draw up an annual plan and review the year as determined by key influencing aspects, such as workload. Also, the team should plan how to monitor and at what point to stop and evaluate. Again, all the staff should be involved at this point in determining timescales and in the auditing process.

Evaluation

The core team needs to establish a formal evaluation process for the information gathered. This involves evaluating care, feeding back and taking action for further evaluation, and may take the form of formal reports, charts or action plans. It needs to be decided:

(1) At what point will information be gathered, and will it be concurrent or retrospective?
(2) Who will collect the information?
(3) Is the relevant information technology available in which to enter and analyse the data?
(4) How often is information gathered/analysed?
(5) Who writes reports?
(6) How will the information be distributed?

Quarterly evaluation needs to be incorporated into the annual plan and the quality team should meet regularly for a continuous assessment of ongoing activity.

It is vital to nurture the underlying principle that the exercise is to identify opportunities to enhance and develop the quality of care and services. It is also important to get rid of the old concept of finding fault, while seeking constantly to improve the total performance of equipment, systems and personnel.

Monitoring and evaluation must eventually lead to the con- clusions, recommendations, actions and follow-up being reported to the appropriate people. The quality team should disseminate information throughout the unit and externally where applicable. A procedure should be established to relay back comments, reactions and information from staff. This should cover, firstly, the effectiveness of the monitoring and evaluation systems used; second, the value of information received; and third, the result of recommendations and action plans. The wider the dissemination of information and feedback the greater the opportunity to benefit from the work.

Annual evaluation

The aspects of care which are chosen for ongoing monitoring should be regularly reviewed and the unit manager is responsible for ensuring an annual report is drawn up and disseminated. This report may assist in drafting the annual business plan for purchasers of care within the unit.

Monitoring tools

Patient satisfaction

First, it is essential to establish what day surgery patients believe they want and then see if it is possible to build those requirements into the service. To do this one should:

- talk to patients and their carers
- use pre- and post-operative screening
- ensure that design of patient surveys is properly researched
- use patients' own language
- monitor trends
- repeat the patient satisfaction audit tool to measure improvements.

Figure 10.1 is an example of some of the language used in a day surgery patient survey.

It is also important to speak to GPs, Community Health Councils, purchasers, district and practice nurses and the general public to find out their conceptions of day surgery, in particular their fears. The results taken from a patients' survey then need to be compared to the unit staff's perceptions of patients' needs and requirements. The differences found will give a picture of the scale of the gap in expectations.

Some patients we have spoken to recently said that they felt unable to ask questions about their surgery and treatment, or about having an anaesthetic and its after-effects.

These patients' comments have been used in the statements below. Please indicate your score of agreement with them.

(Please circle appropriate number)	Strongly agree				Strongly disagree		No opinion/ not applicable
Before my operation I wanted to know the after-effects of the anaesthetic	1	2	3	4	5	6	0
I was told everything I wanted to know about what my surgery/ treatment involved	1	2	3	4	5	6	0
I received good information from the nursing staff about how I would feel after my surgery/treatment	1	2	3	4	5	6	0
I wanted to ask the doctor questions, but it just didn't seem right	1	2	3	4	5	6	0
I was told all of the possible after-effects of having an anaesthetic	1	2	3	4	5	6	0
After seeing the doctor I still felt unsure about some aspects of my treatment	1	2	3	4	5	6	0
I was told everything I wanted to know about the outcome of my operation/ treatment	1	2	3	4	5	6	0
I was not given enough information about the sort of problems to expect after discharge	1	2	3	4	5	6	0

Please add any further comments you may have about information and communication.

_____

_____

Fig. 10.1 Example of the language used in a patient survey. Reproduced with permission of The Patient Survey Unit, United Bristol Healthcare Trust, Bristol Royal Infirmary.

With patients' views as the starting point of change, it is then possible to involve them at all stages of care in planning changes or new services and in the delivery of reviewing and care. This can be done in stages, starting with specific areas of concern and moving on to others later. It is important to re-examine concerns later to ensure such problems do not reoccur.

The nursing process

The nursing process is a systematic analytical approach to patient care.

Dorthea Orem's care planning process (Nursing Models and Nursing Process) applies well to the day surgery patient in that it encourages nurses to act in a complimentary way with patients and families in order to enable self care to be achieved. Monitoring the effectiveness of that process involves many indicators, including audit of the actual care plan, patient surveys and the staff development programme. The use of information from any one of these in isolation does not give a complete record.

Audit of care plans

The process of planning care in day surgery usually takes place prior to admission and care plans may be started at the pre-admission visit. This care continues through surgical preparation, intervention, recovery and discharge. In many units the care plan only ends with the post-discharge telephone follow-up.

Part of the assessment of delivery of care is to monitor how systematic delivery of planned care is assessed and recorded. This will take the form of monitoring various aspects of care in each area (see Figs 10.2, 10.3 and 10.4).

To run the plan one simply audits the completeness of the care plan concurrently with other indicators. This could be with a continuous monitoring process or by using 'snapshot' information taken at random times, and may be undertaken by an external assessor. In most day surgery units, nursing staff are responsible for the design of the day surgery care plan and it is important that they are also responsible for designing and implementing the quality assurance tool to monitor that care. However, monitoring how a care plan is completed can only be part of the total auditing process of the effectiveness of patient care delivery.

Pre-operative	Yes	No	NA	If not, why not
Patient followed pre-op instructions				
Consent form signed				
Arrangements made for discharge				
Allergies recorded				
Relevant medical history recorded				
Admission time recorded				
Correct checking procedure into theatre, i.e. wristband site marked				
Patient assessment complete	Comment:			
Named nurse signature				
. . . .				

Fig. 10.2 Indicator of completeness of the care plan: pre-operative.

Operating theatre/Anaesthetic RM	Yes	No	NA	If not, why not
Time into theatre				
Operation performed noted				
Swabs/instruments/sharps counted				
Position of patient recorded				
Diathermy type/position				
Tourniquet – when on/off				
Dressings – type				
Sutures – type				
Drains – where/type				
Specimens dealt with				
Type of anaesthetic shown				
Named nurse signature	Comment:			
. . . .				

Fig. 10.3 Indicator of completeness of the care plan: operating theatre/anaesthetic room.

Recovery/Discharge	Yes	No	NA	If not, why not
Time into recovery				
Airway status				
Wound site status				
Pain level recorded				
Post-op instructions verbal/written				
Medication given/recorded				
Supplies to take home noted				
Discharged into the care of a responsible adult				
Discharge criteria completed				
Discharge time				
Named nurse signature	Comment:			
. . . .				

Fig. 10.4 Indicator of completeness of care plan: recovery/discharge.

Staff development

A bottom-up approach in which nursing staff identify problems and solutions, and implement and evaluate changes, devolves ownership and control to practitioners. This was seen to result in the most positive outcomes for nursing staff when put into practice at the Bristol Day Surgery Unit.

This concept of ownership and control is very much part of the total quality plan and must be concurrent with monitoring staff involvement, development and satisfaction. Widespread staff participation is the basis of the programme. One of the best ways of achieving this is through a systematic training and development programme with each individual monitoring their own professional profile. They must receive encouragement, guidance and support to develop their individual skills and experience, capitalising on strengths and tackling their deficiencies. How this is monitored depends on the performance monitoring system used. However, once established a regular six-monthly review needs to be in place as part of the plan (see Fig. 10.5).

Name of individual:				Grade:
Performance review objectives	Yes	No	NA	If not, why not
Initial performance review achieving in three stages (minimum)				
Quality of care objectives being achieved				
Resource management objectives being achieved				
Personal career development objectives being achieved				
Clinical skill objectives being achieved				
Interpersonal skills management objectives being achieved				
Organisational skills objectives being achieved				
Six-monthly review arranged				
Assessor's signature				

Fig. 10.5   Staff indicator – performance review with clearly defined objectives.

Outcomes monitoring and variance report

The method of gathering statistical information is very much dependent on the resources in each unit. However, detailed variance reports offer invaluable data that can be utilised as part of the programme and can offer vital clinical outcome information. In order to effectively monitor variance it is necessary to know:

- age groups
- types of surgery
- departments within the unit.

It is important to offer a continuous monitoring. This could be through a form attached to the patient's notes/care plan that follows the patient episode, or completed as a daily worksheet for the entire unit (see Figs 10.6, 10.7, 10.8).

Patient name: Patient no:

Operation: Consultant:

Pre-op	Time in	Please ✓
Patient	Patient arrived late Patient did not follow pre-op instructions Other (explain)	
Care giver	Surgeon/anaesthetist arrived late (circle) Consent not completed Site not marked Other (explain)	
System	Patient arrived too early Patient does not meet day surgery criteria Previous case longer than expected Other (explain) Not enough op time/surgeon not available (circle)	

Fig. 10.6   Variance monitoring tool: pre-operative.

	Time in: Start: End:	Please ✓
Patient	Refused treatment Other (explain)	
Care giver	Difficult induction Difficulty in waking patient Other (explain)	
System	Staff shortage Patients X-ray delayed Instrument/equipment not working Theatre/room not ready Other (explain)	

Fig. 10.7   Variance monitoring tool: operating theatre/anaesthetic room.

Time in recovery: _____ Discharge time: _____

		Please √
Patient	No transport home No responsible adult to collect Delay in lift/responsible adult Nausea Hypertension Pain control inadequate Sleepy Unable to pass urine Other (explain)	
Care giver	Waiting for a decision to admit Incomplete post-op instructions Delay in tablets to take home Other (explain)	

Fig. 10.8 Variance monitoring tool: recovery/discharge.

Other monitoring tools

These include hazard surveillance, risk management surveys, infection control questionnaires and resuscitation equipment check-lists. With these safety checks are done and employees are updated to keep the day surgery unit a safe place for employees and patients.

Continuous quality improvement calendar

A unit calendar prepared by the quality assurance day surgery team which maps out when the various monitoring tools are used also records an overview of the outcome (see Fig. 10.9).

Important aspects of care	Evaluation date	Review date	Outcome

Nursing care:
  Documentation – care plan
  Outcomes management
   (variance reports)			

Fig. 10.9 Continuous quality improvement calendar.

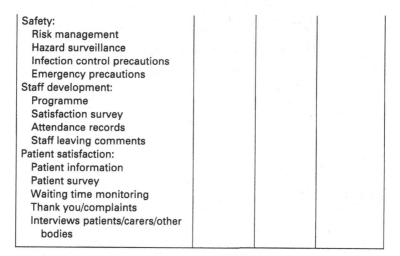

Safety:
  Risk management
  Hazard surveillance
  Infection control precautions
  Emergency precautions
Staff development:
  Programme
  Satisfaction survey
  Attendance records
  Staff leaving comments
Patient satisfaction:
  Patient information
  Patient survey
  Waiting time monitoring
  Thank you/complaints
  Interviews patients/carers/other
    bodies			

Fig. 10.9 Contd.

Key messages

(1) The nursing profession has always aimed for quality care but total quality care is 'an organisation wide meeting of customers needs'.

(2) The study teams must have representatives of all those involved in day care including the patients.

(3) The planning, monitoring and evaluations must be masterminded by those informed in the methods.

(4) Quality controls like audit, risk management and clinical research are only worth the expense if they are first class.

References and further reading

Audit Commission *Measuring Quality: The Patients' View of Day Surgery*, HMSO, London, 1991.

Baldwin, B. *Quality Assurance*, Patient Survey Unit, Bristol Healthcare Trust, 1992.

Munroe-Faure, L.M. *Implementing Total Quality Management*, Pitman Publishing, London, 1992.

National Health Service Management Executive Value-for-Money Unit, *Quality in Action*, HMSO, London, 1993.

Schroeder, R.G. *Operations Management – Decision-Making in the Operations Function*, McGraw Hill, 1989.

Chapter 11
The Way Ahead for Day Surgery

Harold T. Davenport

Introduction

Foreseeing the future in the practice of medicine is a foolhardy habit but nevertheless one that is indulged in widely. Though we expect some censure, we believe that guessing about the direction day surgery may take will lighten our otherwise factual text. Here is the future as we perceive it.

Environment

General practitioners, specialists and consultants may undertake more operating in their offices and clinics using day care organisational arrangements which they will have seen to be so helpful. While most of these operations would be with local anaesthesia, groups of doctors and dentists may well extend their practice to the use of general anaesthetic work. Conversely the convenience, efficient organisation and congeniality of a well-run day care unit can and will attract procedures which are currently scattered across various departments.

Those dentists who have always done local anaesthetic sedation and general anaesthetic work away from hospitals may find that using a day centre is preferable for both them and their patients. Psychiatrists holding electro-convulsive therapy sessions may feel less insecure in a day surgery unit than a ward or clinical side room. Even urgent procedures at present done in accident and emergency departments may be better performed as day cases, so long as they do not disrupt routine work and always involve a trained surgeon. This, like other elective work of the day surgery, would enable better screening of those at risk, particularly young and old, away from the hyperactivity of the out-patient department. Ultimately, acceptance of the enlarged day care complex which will incorporate all non-invasive investigation and therapy may arise through pilot projects such as the one planned at the Central Middlesex Hospital. The experienced day care nurse will be indispensable in all these ventures and venues.

These possibilities are dependent on medico–legal rulings and whether prepaid insurance agencies approve and encourage such developments. The close association of day surgery and day medical units with recovery suites, hospital hotels, parent and carer accommodation and five-day wards which already function should logically flourish.

It has yet to be determined how different these units will be. The form which day care and associated units adopt when freed from hospital design could be remarkably avant-garde. One example for patient entertainment and information – apart from the obvious staff training capabilities – would be the introduction of virtual reality and interactive CD-ROM systems as soon as they evolve. When computer systems are developed which are cheaper, reliable and easily mastered, such information technology will make less arduous the increased productivity of day care.

The content of units must also be much more specifically designed to enable rapid, comfortable and quiet accomplishment of the work in hand. Thus, easy-to-operate trolleys and operating tables plus automatic monitoring and recording apparatus which are so essential to day care will be pioneered here and then used in the hospital in general. Every product required in day care should have its suitability examined and evaluated with the object of producing improvement in patient care and the general efficiency of the unit.

Service development

Since its formation in 1948 the National Health Service has been seen as a government welfare charity type of service, dominated by senior staff and civil servants. The recent momentous reforms have aimed to change it to a patient-demand system, centred in primary health care. Previously, many users looked upon the service as being free at the point of entry and without cost, until recent advances and the rise in expectations made this clearly erroneous.

The new patient and purchaser power could overwhelm day

care if it is not properly handled, and it is therefore essential to control the increase in day surgery by ensuring it is due to developments in preferred clinical practice. This entails much introspection and presentation to a discerning public of the facts, in particular as regards the feasibility of the clinical outcome expected. Politicians must be persuaded that charters or master plans are not really applicable to the vicissitudes of patient care. Patient-representative bodies such as health councils or community voice groups which liaise with hospital trusts can be helpful, but staff advising the public are sometimes the less clinically committed and their message can be prejudicial or misleading. Day care should be straightforward and readily presentable but must be framed so as to be unambiguous.

The success of day care to date presents a major problem in making victims of the staff through overloading with daily diverse expanding workloads. As new tasks arrive they must be assigned the required monies and staff, or else the introduction of new procedures should be postponed. Implementation of expanding day care demands careful and full cooperation with the local GPs and community services. To date their worries about the impact of day care have been unfounded.

As day surgery units handle an increasing number of routine cases, in-patient wards will receive more emergency, major and chronic work, and the effect of this shift needs urgent study. This may require adjustments of both monies and staff distribution. A further problem created by success is the number of visitor-observers the larger day units have been called upon to host. As, and if, this diminishes the energy expended will have to be redirected, to increase the day unit's potential for training and research in new procedures and management. With each new project a proper pilot and then full-blown study is required.

Day care rewards

In simplest terms day care is the best possible provision of secondary care for the majority of patients. In a climate of seemingly overwhelming difficulties within our hospitals a wholesale pessimism and low morale is evident, but with the right backing the day care field has every right to be optimistic and buoyant. If managerial restrictions to day care are proportional to their other financial commitments, it is necessary to explore all other sources of money. Reluctant users of day care who are being pressured by further in-patient limitations have to be made to accept the rules the majority of users have framed. Indeed a great reward that day care can provide to the health service is the solid commitment to the team approach. Modern medicine is so complex and sophisticated it is not achievable by the individual practitioner. The fulfilment provided both professionally and socially each working day by a day care team is enviable.

Key messages

(1) Universal creation of unhospital-like suites for expansion of short stay medicine and surgery is envisaged.
(2) Patient preference plus staff conviction and convenience will make day care the usual practice.
(3) The circumvention of in-hospital strictures and frustrations makes day care a potential delight for patients and staff.

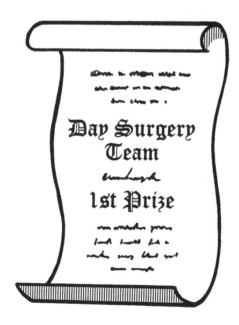

Appendix I

American Society of Anesthesiologists (ASA) new classification of physical status

Class 1

The patient has no organic, physiological, biochemical or psychiatric disturbance. The pathological process for which operation is to be performed is localised and does not entail a systemic disturbance. Examples: a fit patient with inguinal hernia; fibroid uterus in an otherwise healthy woman.

Class 2

Mild to moderate systemic disturbance caused either by the condition to be treated surgically or by other pathophysiological processes. Examples: non- or only slightly limiting organic heart disease, mild diabetes, essential hypertension or anaemia. Some might choose to list the extremes of age here, either the neonate or the octogenerian, even though no discernible systemic disease is present. Extreme obesity and chronic bronchitis may be included in this category.

Class 3

Severe systemic disturbance or disease from whatever cause, even though it may not be possible to define the degree of disability with finality. Examples: severely limiting organic heart disease; severe diabetes with vascular complications; moderate to severe degrees of pulmonary insufficiency; angina pectoris or healed myocardial infarction.

Class 4

Severe systemic disorders that are already life threatening, not always correctable by operation. Examples: patients with organic heart disease showing marked signs of cardiac insufficiency, persistent angina or active myocarditis; advanced degrees of pulmonary, hepatic, renal or endocrine insufficiency.

Class 5

The moribund patient who has little chance of survival but is submitted to operation in desperation. Examples: the burst abdominal aneurysm with profound shock; major cerebral trauma with rapidly increasing intracranial pressure; massive pulmonary embolus. Most of these patients require operation as a resuscitative measure with little if any anaesthesia.

(Original source: *Anesthesiology*, 1963, **24**, p. 111.)

Appendix II

'Pharmacy Services' leaflet
'Your Bed Area' leaflet
'Breast Care Service' leaflet

PHARMACY SERVICES

The hospital pharmacy is situated in the new building in the out-patients department.

Will I need medicines to take home?

If you need medicines to take at home after your procedure, they will usually be given to you from supplies held on the suite at the time you are discharged. However, occasionally medicines are prescribed that are **not** stocked on the day surgery suite. If that happens, we may ask you to collect them from the hospital pharmacy. Follow the sign posts to the out-patients department then look for the sign to pharmacy. You will **not** need to pay for any medicines you take home with you from the day surgery suite.

Will I be given painkillers?

If you are given medicines for pain relief, please make sure you read the information leaflet you are given with the medicine, as it will tell you how to get the best effects from the painkillers. If you take any painkillers regularly (e.g. for arthritis, back pain, headaches, etc.) make sure you tell the nurse **either** when you are admitted **or** before you go home, so we can check whether you should take the painkillers we prescribe **instead of** or **in addition to** what you are taking already.

Should I keep taking the medicines my GP prescribes?

We asked you to bring all the medicines that you take regularly into hospital with you. While you are staying on the day surgery suite please continue to take your medicines as you would at home **unless** the doctor or nurse who admitted you has told you not to.

If you are not sure whether or not you need to take your regular medicines **please ask a nurse** and they will find out what you should do.

Who can I ask if I have some more questions about my medicines after leaving hospital?

If you would like to ask any questions about the medicines you take regularly or the medicines you are given after your procedure, please telephone the pharmacy drug information department between 9am and 5pm and ask to speak to a pharmacist. We are always happy to help.

YOUR BED AREA

Each patient area is designed to meet your needs for comfort and convenience during your stay. Your bed/trolley is made as a pre-operative bed, i.e. a ready-made bed for patients going to theatre. If, however, you find that this is insufficient or you feel too cold, please do not hesitate to ask the ward staff for extra blankets, etc.

A locker is provided for your personal belongings. We do ask that prior to going to theatre you use the cupboards and drawers and leave your bed area tidy.

An overhead lamp is attached to the wall which can be angled to meet your needs, and dimmed if required by flicking the switch on the wall. Nursing staff will be happy to give assistance where required.

You will also have a table for you to use around the bed area which can be raised or lowered depending on individual need. Again the ward staff will show you how this is done.

Each bed area has a nurse-call button. This is for use when requiring assistance from one of the nursing staff, and enables nurses to react quickly to your needs.

BREAST CARE SERVICE

The Kent and Canterbury Hospital Breast Care Service offers help, information and support to women with breast cancer or other breast related problems. Its services include:

- Access to a specialist breast care nurse.
- A range of information leaflets on aspects of breast care and treatment including support services.
- A sensitive and complete breast prosthesis fitting service (by appointment only).

Help and information

The specialist breast care nurse can answer your and your family's questions about treatments for non-cancerous breast conditions and breast cancer. This includes possible side effects and any medical problems you may be experiencing.

Emotional support and understanding

Emotional difficulties linked to cancer are not always easy to talk about and are often hardest to share with those to whom you are closest. Talking to the breast care nurse may provide the support you are seeking, she can also introduce you to a volunteer who has breast cancer or to a local cancer support group.

If you have any questions or would like help with practical problems and need support, contact:

Name
Breast care nurse specialist
Tel no.

- Breast prostheses are available free on the NHS.
- A good selection of prostheses and bras are available for you to try on with assistance from an experienced fitter.
- Advice on how to adapt your existing wardrobe, choosing clothes and swimwear.
- Bras may be purchased at a very reasonable price.

This is a personal and confidential service. We must, therefore, ask you to telephone for an appointment. If you wish to make an appointment, please contact:

Name, Tel no.

Appendix III

'Laparoscopic Hernia' patient
information leaflet

'Cardioversion' patient information
leaflet

'Breast Localisation and Removal of
Breast Lump' patient information
leaflet

Information For You About Your Operation

LAPAROSCOPIC HERNIA (Rupture) Repair

Day/Short Stay Services

Welcome to your ward

The following notes contain information which we hope will answer questions you may have regarding your operation for *Laparoscopic Hernia (Rupture) Repair*. The operation is performed by using a 'telescope' like instrument and therefore necessitates only a short stay in hospital.

Before your admission day – meeting your nurse

You have been asked to come to the ward on a day before your operation to see your nurse so that he/she can obtain your medical history. The doctor may also examine you. Any investigations necessary at this time will be arranged, e.g. blood tests. It is very important that you remember to tell the nurse about any serious illnesses/operations that you have had in the past; if in doubt tell the nurse. You should also mention any tablets or medicines you are taking. Also if you are allergic to any tablets, medicines, tapes or plasters. Be prepared to spend one hour at the hospital. Before your admission, if necessary, the area on which you are going to have your operation will need to be shaved. Shave all hair growth on your abdomen (tummy). Please do this at home *on your admission day*.

Admission day

Please ensure that you arrive at the time shown in your admission letter. If your admission time is before 11 am you will have your operation during the morning. If it is at 11 am your operation will be in the afternoon.

It is very important that you *do not have anything to eat or drink* after the time shown in your letter. If you are taking regular medicines you may take them at the usual time with the smallest amount of water (unless you have been told otherwise). Remember to bring your medicines with you.

Arrival at the day surgery suite

The receptionist will greet you when you arrive and show you to your bed. If the receptionist is not available please wait on the seats outside the ward. Your nurse will then introduce her/himself and ask you some questions and help you to prepare for going to theatre. You will be asked to remove all clothing and put on a white gown. The doctor may come and see you. When you are due to go to theatre you will be taken (on either a bed or trolley) by two hospital porters and your nurse. You will be greeted in theatre by the reception nurse who is responsible for your care until you are taken into the anaesthetic room. Here you will meet the anaesthetist who will give you an injection into the back of the hand which will put you to sleep.

After your operation – pain relief

You will wake up in the recovery ward (your operation is now over). If you experience any discomfort or pain on return to the ward the nursing staff will give you tablets or an injection. Some people experience pain in the shoulder following this procedure. This is due to insertion of gas during the operation. This is quite normal. Please ask the nurse for painkillers.

Your operation – time in hospital

Expect to stay in hospital for the rest of the day. You will have four small plasters covering the wounds. These may be changed before you are discharged.

Initially you will feel drowsy and might feel sick. Once this has passed you will be allowed out of bed, to sit in a chair. When you feel more able you can walk to the toilet, with assistance if necessary. Sandwiches, tea and coffee are available at any time when you feel able to eat and drink. When you are mobile with little discomfort and have passed urine, you may be discharged home.

When you go home

You must have someone to accompany you home. *DO NOT* use public transport. The doctor may see you before you go home. You will be given a supply of painkillers and a letter addressed to your GP. This is to tell him/her of your operation and should be *handed in at your surgery within 24 hours*. An appointment will be made with your GP's surgery for removal of your stitches if this is necessary.

Your dressings should be left untouched for 48 hours after which time they can be removed and you may take a shower or bath. The wounds should look clean and healed; if there is any redness or oozing or if you are at all worried, contact your GP's surgery for advice.

For the first few days after your operation you will feel weak and tired and need help to do the household chores. Whatever type of operation you have had, during the first week to 10 days at home, you may feel weak, tired and a little depressed. We call this 'post-operative blues'. This will pass but if symptoms persist, please consult your GP for help and advice.

You should not stay in bed and it is important that you 'potter about' until you feel stronger and able to do more. You *should not do any heavy lifting or heavy manual work* until you are comfortable to do so or for two months, whichever is shorter. This includes 'digging the garden'! You should refrain from work for two weeks or until your GP is happy for your return. You may drive a car after your stitches have been removed if you feel confident and are able to do an emergency stop.

Normal sexual relations may be resumed once you feel comfortable to do so.

Do not drink alcohol for 24 hours after your operation.

Diet

After your operation you may eat normally. There are no restrictions on your diet. However, some people experience constipation. You should drink at least two litres of fluid a day for the first two to three days. Please consult your GP for advice should constipation occur.

Tablets and medicines

You may continue to take your tablets and medicines as normal unless given instructions to the contrary. Pain killing tablets should be taken regularly for the first 48 hours. *Do not* wait until the pain is unbearable.

If you wish to be treated privately we can provide single rooms with en suite facilities. Please ring to discuss arrangements.

We hope that we have been able to answer some of your questions. If you require any more information please do not hesitate to ask us either before or after your operation. Please ring and your nurse will be only too happy to help. We all wish you a speedy recovery following your operation.

Summary

Your operation is for Laparoscopic Hernia (Rupture) Repair

Before your admission day

You will come to the ward to see the nurse
You may undergo some tests
Be prepared to spend one hour at the hospital

On the day

Arrive on time
Do not eat or drink after the stated time
Shave the operation area
Take your usual medicines (unless told otherwise)
Bring any regular medication with you

After your operation

You will be given medication for relief of pain; take regularly
Your dressings may be changed before you go home
You may be seen by a doctor
Arrangements will be made to have any stitches removed, if necessary
You may be given a letter for your GP
Arrange for someone to take you home

At home

You will need help with the household chores
Remember to keep the dressings dry for 48 hours
Check wounds after 48 hours, then bath/shower
No heavy lifting or manual work until comfortable
No driving until stitches have been removed and you feel able to do an emergency stop
Normal sexual relations when comfortable
Return to work when your GP allows

After reading this information, are there any questions you would like to ask? Please list below and ask your nurse:

_____

_____

_____

_____

Information For You About Your Treatment

CARDIOVERSION

Day/Short Stay Services

Welcome to your ward

The following notes contain information which we hope will answer questions you may have regarding your admission for *Cardioversion*.

Your doctor has found that your heart beat is irregular, in technical terms, known as atrial fibrillation (AF). It is often possible to put your heart back to the usual regular rhythm with cardioversion. This is not an operation, but does require a light anaesthetic. While you are anaesthetised, a doctor will administer an electric shock to the chest and heart, which, if successful, will reset the rhythm of the heart so that it becomes regular. Following recovery from the anaesthetic you will be allowed home as described below. There is minimal discomfort, although some people do find that the skin over the chest is a little sore for a day or so. Unfortunately, the procedure is not always successful, in which case the doctor will treat you appropriately.

Before your admission day – meeting the doctor and your nurse

You have been asked to come to the ward on a day before your cardioversion to see the nurse and, if necessary, the doctor so he/she can obtain your medical history. Any investigations necessary at this time will be arranged, e.g. blood tests. It is very important that you remember to tell the nurse about any serious illnesses/operations that you have had in the past; if in any doubt tell the nurse. You should mention any tablets or medicines you are taking, also if you are allergic to any tablets, medicines, tapes or plasters. We would hope these procedures will take no longer than one hour.

Admission day

Please ensure that you arrive at the time shown in your admission letter.

It is very important that you *do not have anything to eat or drink* after the time shown in your letter. If you are taking regular medicines you may take them at the usual time with the smallest amount of water (unless you have been told otherwise). Remember to bring your medicines with you.

Arrival at the day surgery suite

The receptionist will greet you when you arrive at reception and show you to your bed. If the receptionist is not available please wait on the seats outside reception. Your nurse will then introduce her/himself and ask you some questions and help you to prepare for going to theatre. You will be asked to remove all clothing and put on a white gown. When you are due to go to theatre you will be taken (on either a bed or trolley) by two hospital porters and your nurse. You will be greeted in theatre by the reception nurse who is responsible for your care until you are taken into the anaesthetic room. Here you will meet the anaesthetist who will give you an injection into the back of the hand which will put you to sleep.

After your cardioversion – pain relief

You will wake up in the recovery ward (your cardioversion is now over). If you experience any discomfort or pain on return to the ward the nursing staff will give you tablets to relieve this.

Your cardioversion – time in hospital

Expect to stay in hospital for the rest of the day.

Initially you will feel drowsy and might feel sick. Once this has passed you will be allowed out of bed, to sit in a chair. When you feel more able you can walk to the toilet, with assistance if necessary. Sandwiches, tea and coffee are available at any time when you feel able to eat and drink.

You will have an ECG (a tracing of the heart) before you leave the ward.

Whatever type of operation/procedure you have had, during the first week to 10 days at home, you may feel weak, tired and a little depressed. We call this 'post-operative blues'. This will pass but if symptoms persist, please consult your GP for help and advice.

When you go home

You must have someone to accompany you home. *DO NOT* use public transport. The doctor may see you before you go home. You may also be given a letter addressed to your GP. This is to tell him/her of your treatment and should be *handed in at your surgery within 24 hours.*

You should have a responsible adult at home with you for the first 24 hours.

Diet

After your cardioversion you may eat normally. There are no restrictions on your diet.

Tablets and medicines

You may continue to take your tablets and medicines as normal unless given instructions to the contrary.

If you wish to be treated privately we can provide single rooms with en suite facilities. Please ring to discuss arrangements.

We hope that we have been able to answer some of your questions. If you require any more information please do not hesitate to ask us either before or after your operation. Please ring and your nurse will be only too happy to help. We all wish you a speedy recovery following your cardioversion.

Summary

Your cardioversion
Your admission is for Cardioversion

Before your admission day

You will come to the ward to see the nurse
You may undergo some tests
Be prepared to spend one hour at the hospital

On the day

Arrive on time
Do not eat or drink after the stated time
Take your usual medicines (unless told otherwise)
Bring any regular medication with you

After your cardioversion

You may be seen by a doctor
You will be given a letter for your GP
Arrange for someone to take you home
You will have an ECG

At home

You should resume normal activities the following day

After reading this information, are there any questions you would like to ask? Please list below and ask your nurse:

_____

_____

_____

_____

Information For You About Your Operation

BREAST LOCALISATION and REMOVAL OF BREAST LUMP

Day/Short Stay Services

Welcome to your ward

The following notes contain information which we hope will answer some of the questions you may have regarding your *Breast Localisation followed by Removal of a Breast Lump*. Breast localisation will take place in the breast screening unit. This is where a fine wire is inserted into the breast. This wire is removed, with the breast lump, later, by the surgeon.

Before your admission day – meeting your nurse

You have been asked to come to the ward on a day before your operation to see your nurse so that he/she can obtain your medical history. The doctor may also examine you. Any investigations necessary at this time will be arranged, e.g. blood tests. It is very important that you remember to tell the nurse about any serious illnesses/operations that you have had in the past; if in doubt tell the nurse. You should also mention any tablets or medicines you are taking. Also if you are allergic to any tablets, medicines, tapes or plasters. We would hope these procedures will take no longer than one hour. The breast care nurse specialist is available for support and advice, and can be contacted on ....

Admission day

Please ensure that you arrive at the time shown in your admission letter. If your admission time is before 11.00 am you will have your operation during the morning. If it is 11.00 am your operation will be in the afternoon.

It is very important that you *do not have anything to eat or drink* after the time shown in your letter. If you are taking regular medicines you may take them at the usual time with the smallest amount of water (unless you have been told otherwise). Remember to bring your medicines with you.

Arrival at the day surgery suite

The receptionist will greet you when you arrive and show you to your bed/trolley. If the receptionist is not available please wait on the seats outside the ward. Your nurse will then introduce her/himself and ask you some questions and help you to prepare for your procedure. The doctor may also see you. During the morning you will be taken on your bed to the breast screening unit. Here you will have a mammogram which will show the exact area of your breast lump/abnormal area. After the mammogram a small needle will be inserted into this area. The needle will then be left in place. Prior to this you will have been given some local anaesthetic into the skin (this injection does sting). You will return to the ward. When you are due to go to theatre you will be taken (on either a bed or trolley) by two hospital porters and your nurse. You will be greeted in theatre by the reception nurse who is responsible for your care until you are taken into the anaesthetic room. Here you will meet the anaesthetist who will give you an injection into the back of the hand which will put you to sleep.

After your operation – pain relief

You will wake up in the recovery ward (your operation is now over). If you experience any discomfort or pain on return to the ward the nursing staff will give you tablets or an injection to relieve this.

Your operation – time in hospital

Expect to stay in hospital for the rest of the day (or overnight if it is necessary).

You will have a dressing covering the wound, this may be changed before you are discharged. You may find it comfortable to wear a bra after your operation. This is not essential.

If you have a drain in the wound (this is a plastic tube leading into a bottle, to collect any drainage from the wound) this will be removed before you go home.

Initially you will feel drowsy and may feel sick. Once this has passed you will be allowed out of bed, to sit in a chair. When you feel more able you can walk to the toilet, with assistance if necessary.

Sandwiches, tea and coffee are available at any time when you feel able to eat and drink.

When you go home

You *must* have someone to accompany you home. *Do not* use public transport. The doctor may see you before you go home. You will be given a supply of painkillers and may be given a letter addressed to your GP. This is to tell him of your operation and should be *handed in at your surgery within 24 hours*. An appointment will be made with your GP's surgery for removal of your stitches. This is usually one week after the operation. Your dressing should be left untouched for 48 hours. The dressing can then be removed and you may take a shower or bath. The wound should look clean and healed, if there is any redness or oozing or if you are at all worried, contact your GP's surgery for advice. An out-patient appointment (if necessary) will be given. Initially when you go home you may feel tired and weak and will need help with the household chores.

Whatever type of operation you have had, during the first week to 10 days at home, you may feel weak, tired and a little depressed. We call this 'post-operative blues'. This will pass but if symptoms persist, please consult your GP for help and advice.

You should have a responsible adult at home with you for the first 24 hours.

You should refrain from work until your stitches have been removed or until your GP is happy for your return. You may drive a car when you are confident to do an emergency stop.

Normal sexual relations may be resumed once you feel comfortable to do so.

Do not cook, drink alcohol or drive for 24 hours after your operation.

Diet

There are no restrictions on your diet. You may eat and drink normally.

Tablets and medicines

You may continue to take your tablets and medicines as normal unless given instructions to the contrary. Take painkillers regularly. Do not wait until the pain becomes unbearable.

If you wish to be treated privately we can provide single rooms with en suite facilities. Please ring .... to discuss arrangements.

We hope that we have been able to answer some of your questions. If you require any more information please do not hesitate to ask us either before or after your operation. Please ring .... where your nurse will be only too happy to help. We all wish you a speedy recovery following your operation.

Summary

Your operation is breast localisation/excision breast lump.

Before your admission day

You will come to the ward to see the nurse
You may undergo some tests
Be prepared to spend one hour at the hospital

On the day

Arrive on time
Do not eat or drink after the stated time
Take your usual medicines (unless told otherwise)
Bring any regular medication with you

After your operation

You will be given medication for relief of pain; take regularly
Your dressing may be changed before you go home
You may be seen by a doctor
Arrangements will be made to have your stitches removed
You may be given a letter for your GP
Arrange for someone to take you home

At home

You will need help with the household chores
Check wound after 48 hours
No driving until stitches have been removed and you feel able to do an emergency stop
Normal sexual relations when comfortable
Return to work when your GP allows
Do not drink alcohol or cook for 24 hours

After reading this information, are there any questions you would like to ask? Please list below and ask your nurse:

_____

_____

_____

_____

Appendix IV
'Painkillers' patient information leaflet

Information for you about getting the best from your painkillers

Day/Short Stay Services

Welcome to your ward

Pain relief after your surgery or procedure

Most people suffer pain or discomfort after their surgery. Although we cannot say exactly how you will feel after your surgery, we do know how much pain is felt by most people who have had your kind of operation. So, when you are discharged, the nursing staff will give you the type of painkiller we believe will suit you best. This will be one of three medicines:

- Paracetamol tablets
- Codydramol tablets
- Tylex capsules

Please follow these general instructions to get the best effect from your painkiller. If you have been given Coydramol tablets or Tylex capsules, please read the special section that applies to your medicine.

Getting the best effects from your painkillers

1. For the first 24 hours after surgery

Take the dose of painkillers regularly every six hours whether you have pain or not. Take a dose of ONE or TWO tablets or capsules depending on how you feel. The most important thing is to take the dose regularly. If you decide to take ONE capsule or tablet and you still have pain, take TWO for the next dose. If you still have pain when you are taking TWO every SIX hours tell the nurse from the day surgery unit when she phones, and she will advise you what to do. Never take more than EIGHT tablets or capsules in ONE day (24 hours).

    If you are over 70 years old and have been given Tylex or Codydramol tablets, read the extra information on these medicines before you decide what dose to take.

2. On the second day after surgery

Take ONE or TWO capsules every eight hours (that is, a maximum of six tablets or capsules in 24 hours). However, if you still have pain take the tablets or capsules as you did on day one, that is, every six hours (or a maximum of eight in 24 hours).

3. From the third day after surgery onwards

If you have any pain, take PARACETAMOL TABLETS (available from chemists and shops selling medicines). Follow the instructions on the bottle/packet and do not take more than eight tablets every 24 hours. If this does not control the pain, contact your GP's surgery.

What if the pain is very bad?

If you still have bad pain, even though you are following these instructions, either telephone the day surgery suite and ask for advice, or contact your GP's surgery. Be ready to tell whoever answers the phone what operation or procedure you had and what painkillers you are taking.

Can I take other painkillers as well?

NO!

Do not take any other painkillers without asking your doctor or pharmacist (chemist). Many painkillers contain Paracetamol and/or Codeine. It is dangerous to take more than eight tablets/capsules containing Paracetamol.

Can I take any other medicines?

Keep taking all the medicines you are prescribed by your GP unless you were told **not** to by staff on the day surgery unit. If you usually take painkillers prescribed by your GP which contain Paracetamol (e.g. Co-Codamol, Co-Proxamol, Distalgesic, Solpadeine) you must **not** take these tablets **as well as** the medicines we have given you for your pain.

If you are unsure whether or not you can take any medicines you have at home contact the hospital pharmacy department (tel. XXXX), if it is between the hours of 9am and 5.30pm. Please have your regular medicines handy, so you can read out what they contain.

Some extra information about Tylex capsules and Codydramol tablets

What do they contain?

Tylex capsules each contain Paracetamol 500mg and Codeine 30mg. They are prescribed for moderate to severe pain. DO NOT take Tylex if you think you are allergic to Codeine.

Codydramol tablets each contain Paracetamol 500mg and Dihydro-codeine 10mg. They are prescribed for moderate pain. DO NOT take Codydramol tablets if you think you are allergic to Dihydrocodeine.

Can they cause any side effects?

Both medicines are good at controlling pain but they can cause a number of side effects. They can make you feel dizzy, lightheaded or sleepy, or they can make you feel sick or short of breath. These side effects can all be made worse by moving, so if you feel any of these effects try lying down and resting.

Tylex and Codydramol can also make you constipated. This is not usually a problem when you only take them for a couple of days, but if it is, ask your pharmacist (chemist) to recommend a laxative.

Very rarely, people can suffer an allergic reaction to Tylex or Cody-dramol. They may come out in a rash, feel very short of breath, get swelling of the face or body, or a mixture of these symptoms. If this should happen to you, STOP taking the medicine and telephone your GP straight away for advice on what to do.

If you suffer from asthma you should NOT take these tablets during an acute attack of wheezing, as they can slow your rate of breathing.

Should I take one or two?

People who are over 70 tend to be more likely to suffer from the side effects of these painkillers, so if you are aged 70, and you do not usually take strong painkillers, try a dose of ONE rather than TWO. If you still have pain after 45 minutes take ONE more, then continue taking a dose of TWO every six hours. Try and rest after you have taken a dose and if you need to move about, take extra care.

Finally,

- DON'T drink alcohol while you are taking Tylex or Codydramol.
- DON'T drive or do anything that needs a lot of concentration if you feel dizzy or lightheaded.
- NEVER take more than eight tablets or capsules in 24 hours.

Some general information about medicines

- Always read the label carefully and take the medicine exactly as prescribed.
- Keep your medicine bottles tightly closed and stored in a cool dry place which is WELL OUT OF CHILDREN'S REACH!
- Although your bottle may have a safety top, it does NOT mean that children can't open it. If you can't manage to open the safety cap on your bottle ask the pharmacist (chemist) for an ordinary top. Don't leave your bottles open all the time.
- Never mix different medicines in the same bottle or transfer medicines from one bottle to another. It is very dangerous.
- Never share your medicines with anyone else. They have been chosen especially for you and may harm someone else, even if that person seems to have the same illness.
- If you are told to stop taking a medicine, take any that is left over back to your chemist or flush it down the toilet. Medicines do not keep well and if you need the same drug again a new supply will be given.

REMEMBER
Keep all drugs well out of children's reach
Don't keep drugs you don't use.

Index